Workbook to Accompany
Delmar's Dental Assisting:
A Comprehensive Approach

Workbook to Accompany Delmar's Dental Assisting: A Comprehensive Approach

KAREN WAIDE, CDA, EFDA, AAS
Portland Community College
Portland, Oregon

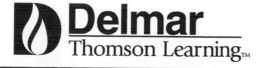

Africa • Australia • Canada • Denmark • Japan • Mexico • New Zealand • Philippines
Puerto Rico • Singapore • Spain • United Kingdom • United States

NOTICE TO THE READER

Publisher does not warrant or guarantee any of the products described herein or perform any independent analysis in connection with any of the product information contained herein. Publisher does not assume, and expressly disclaims, any obligation to obtain and include information other than that provided to it by the manufacturer. The reader is expressly warned to consider and adopt all safety precautions that might be indicated by the activities herein and to avoid all potential hazards. By following the instructions contained herein, the reader willingly assumes all risks in connection with such instructions.

The Publisher makes no representation or warranties of any kind, including but not limited to, the warranties of fitness for particular purpose or merchantability, nor are any such representations implied with respect to the material set forth herein, and the publisher takes no responsibility with respect to such material. The publisher shall not be liable for any special, consequential, or exemplary damages resulting, in whole or part, from the readers' use of, or reliance upon, this material.

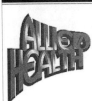
COPYRIGHT © 2000
Delmar is a division of Thomson Learning.
The Thomson Learning logo is a registered trademark
used herein under license.

Printed in Canada
1 2 3 4 5 6 7 8 9 10 XXX 04 03 02 01 00 99

For more information, contact Delmar, 3 Columbia Circle, PO Box 15015, Albany, NY 12212-0515;
or find us on the World Wide Web at http://www.delmar.com

Library of Congress Card No. 98-55682

ISBN: 0-8273-9085-8

Contents

To the Learner

This workbook is designed to accompany *Delmar's Dental Assisting: A Comprehensive Approach*. Using the textbook and this workbook along with other components of Delmar's complete learning system, will help you become a successful dental assistant. Utilizing the complete learning system will help reinforce all of the essential competencies you will need to enter the field of dental assisting and become a highly skilled professional in today's multiskilled health care environment. In addition, this workbook will challenge you to apply basic skills, use assessment evaluations, and integrate your knowledge effectively.

WORKBOOK ORGANIZATION

Workbook chapters are divided into the following sections: Objectives, Summary, Key Terms, Exercises and Activities, and Skill Competency Assessments.

Objectives

The list of objectives reiterates those found at the beginning of each textbook chapter. Reviewing these objectives will reinforce the facts and principles that need to be understood in each chapter.

Summary

Provides a brief overview of the chapter content and describes the responsibilities of the dental assistant.

Key Terms

The key term list serves as a review of the important terminology surrounding the chapter content.

Exercise and Activities

These exercises cover the basic chapter content and terminology, further reinforcing and applying your understanding of the chapter objectives and key terms.

Skill Competency Assessments

This workbook provides Skill Competency Assessment checklist sheets that are designed to correlate with specific information and procedures found in *Delmar's Dental Assisting: A Comprehensive Approach*.

    The checklists are designed to set criteria or standards that should be observed while a specific procedure is performed. They follow the same procedural steps as listed in the textbook. As you perform each procedure the evaluation sections of the sheet are used to judge your performance with an opportunity for self evaluation and student evaluation. The instructor will use this sheet to evaluate your competency in performing the specific skill identified in each procedure. The comment portion of the checklist allows for constructive feedback.

The Skill Competency Assessment sheet is organized as follows:

- *Skill*—describes the procedure.
- *Performance Objective*—identifies what must be successfully demonstrated by the student.
- *Icons*—indicates which function, instruments, and protective equipment are required for the procedure.
- *Equipment and Supplies*—lists the equipment and supplies to be gathered to perform the procedure along with the possible points earned for successfully gathering each piece.
- *Competency Steps*—lists each step to be described or performed by the student in order to successfully complete the procedure along with the possible points earned for completing each step.
- *Total Points*—lists the total points possible for a first or second attempt at performing the procedure along with a space for entering the actual points earned.

The points assigned to each step reflect the importance of that step in meeting the performance objective. An important step is valued with 1 point, an essential step with 2 points, and a critical step with 3 points. Failure results if any of the critical steps are missed or performed incorrectly.

A Skills Tracking sheet is provided on pages ix–xi to serve as a table of contents for all assessments, as well as a guide to easily view your performance.

Be sure to visit Delmar's website for additional Skill Competency Assessment sheets at www.delmaralliedhealth.com/dental.

GENERAL STUDY TIPS

Here are some tips to help you learn more effectively:

- Feel certain that each procedure and concept you master is an important step toward preparing your skills and knowledge for the workplace. The textbook, workbook, and instructor materials have all been coordinated to meet the core objectives. Review the Objectives before you begin to study as they are a road map that will take you to your goal.

- Remember that you are the learner, so you can take credit for your success. The instructor is an important guide on this journey, and the textbook, workbook, and clinical experiences are tools. Whether or not you use these tools wisely is ultimately up to you.

- Evaluate yourself and your study habits. Take positive action toward improving yourself, and avoid habits that could limit your success. For example, do you let family responsibilities or social opportunities interfere with your study? If so, sit down with your family and plan a schedule for study that they will support and to which you will adhere. Find a special place to study that is free from distraction.

Because regulations vary from state to state regarding which procedures can be performed by a dental assistant, it will be important to check specific regulations in your state. A dental assistant should never perform any procedure without being aware of legal responsibilities, correct procedure, and proper authorization.

Enjoy your new career in dental assisting!

SKILLS COMPETENCY ASSESSMENT TRACKING SHEET

Assessment No. and Title	Workbook Page No.	Date Assessment completed & Competency Achieved		
		Self Evaluation Date/Initials	Student Evaluation Date/Initials	Instructor Evaluation Date/Initials
2-1 Applying Disclosing Agent for Plaque Identification	7			
2-2 Bass or Modified Bass Brushing Technique	8			
2-3 Dental Flossing Technique	9			
2-4 Fluoride Application	11			
9-1 Handwashing	40			
9-2 Preparing the Dental Treatment Room	41			
9-3 Completion of Dental Treatment	42			
9-4 Final Treatment Room Disinfecting and Cleaning	44			
9-5 Treatment of Contaminated Tray in the Sterilization Center	45			
11-1 Taking a Radial Pulse and Measuring the Respiration Rate	54			
11-2 Measuring Blood Pressure	55			
13-1 Administration of Oxygen	64			
13-2 Treatment of a Patient with Syncope	65			
14-1 Seating the Dental Patient	69			
14-2 Dismissing the Dental Patient	71			
14-3 One-Handed Instrument Transfer	73			
14-4 Specific Tip Placements for Evacuation of the Oral Cavity	75			
16-1 Preparing the Anesthetic Syringe	84			
16-2 Assisting with the Administration of Topical and Local Anesthetics	86			
17-1 Radiography Infection Control	93			
17-2 Full-Mouth X-Ray Exposure with Paralleling Technique	95			
17-3 Exposing Occlusal Radiographs	97			
17-4 Processing Radiographs Using a Manual Tank	99			
17-5 Processing Radiographs Using an Automatic Processor	101			
17-6 Processing Duplicating Technique	102			
17-7 Mounting Radiographs	103			
18-1 Electronic Pulp Testing	107			
18-2 Root Canal Treatment	108			
19-1 Surgical Scrub	115			
19-2 Multiple Extractions and Alveoplasty	116			
19-3 Removal of Impacted Third Molars	119			
19-4 Treatment for Alveolitis	121			
21-1 Placement and Removal of Elastic Separators	130			
21-2 Cementation of Orthodontic Bands	132			
21-3 Direct Bonding of Brackets	134			
21-4 Placement of the Arch Wire and Ligature Ties	136			
21-5 Completion Appointment	138			

SKILLS COMPETENCY ASSESSMENT TRACKING SHEET *Continued*

Assessment No. and Title	Date Assessment completed & Competency Achieved			
	Workbook Page No.	Self Evaluation Date/Initials	Student Evaluation Date/Initials	Instructor Evaluation Date/Initials
22-1 T-Band Placement	143			
22-2 Pulpotomy	145			
23-1 Scaling, Curettage, and Polishing	150			
23-2 Gingivectomy	152			
23-3 Preparation and Placement of the Non-Eugenol Periodontal Dressing	154			
24-1 Porcelain Veneers	158			
24-2 Preparation for a Porcelain-Fused-to-Metal Crown	162			
24-3 Cementation of Porcelain-Fused-to-Metal Crown	166			
25-1 Final Impression Appointment	171			
25-2 Jaw Relationship Appointment	173			
25-3 The Try-In Appointment	175			
25-4 Denture Relining	177			
26-1 Mixing Zinc Phosphate Cement	182			
26-2 Mixing Zinc Oxide Eugenol Cement— Powder/Liquid Form	184			
26-3 Mixing Polycarboxylate Cement	186			
26-4 Mixing Glass Ionomer Cement	188			
26-5 Mixing of Calcium Hydroxide Cement— Two-Paste System	190			
26-6 Placing Resin Cement—Dual-Curing Technique	191			
26-7 Placing Etchant	193			
26-8 Placing Bonding Agent	194			
26-9 Amalgam Restoration—Class II	196			
26-10 Composite Restoration—Class III	200			
27-1 Preparing for an Alginate Impression	208			
27-2 Taking an Alginate Impression	210			
27-3 Removing the Alginate Impression	212			
27-4 Disinfecting Alginate Impresssions	214			
27-5 Taking a Bite Registration	215			
27-6 Taking a Polysulfide Impresssion	217			
27-7 Pouring an Alginate Impression for a Study Model	219			
27-8 Trimming Diagnostic Casts/Study Models	221			
27-9 Constructing a Self-Cured Acrylic Resin Custom Tray	224			
27-10 Constructing a Vacuum-Formed Acrylic Resin Custom Tray	227			
27-11 Sizing, Adapting, and Seating a Preformed Acrylic Crown	229			
27-12 Adapting, Trimming, and Seating a Matrix and Custom Temporary Restoration	231			
27-13 Cementing the Custom Self-Curing Composite Temporary Crown	233			

SKILLS COMPETENCY ASSESSMENT TRACKING SHEET *Continued*

Assessment No. and Title	Workbook Page No.	Date Assessment completed & Competency Achieved		
		Self Evaluation Date/Initials	Student Evaluation Date/Initials	Instructor Evaluation Date/Initials
28-1 Placing and Removing the Dental Dam	238			
28-2 Assembly of the Tofflemire Matrix	241			
28-3 Coronal Polish	243			
28-4 Placing Cavity Liners	246			
28-5 Placement of Cement Bases	248			
28-6 Removal of the Simple Suture and Continuous Simple Sutures	250			
28-7 Placing and Removing the Retraction Cord	251			
28-8 Placing Enamel Sealants	253			
28-9 In-Office Bleaching for Vital Teeth	256			
29-1 Balancing the Day Sheets and the End-of-the-Month Figures	261			
29-2 Preparing a Deposit Slip	263			
29-3 Reordering Supplies	265			
29-4 Reconciling a Bank Statement	267			

Introduction to the Dental Profession

OBJECTIVES

The student should strive to meet the following objectives and demonstrate an understanding of the facts and principles presented in this chapter:

1. Identify oral disease indications from the beginning of time.
2. List the names of individuals who had a great impact on the profession of dentistry.
3. Identify the people who promoted education and organized dentistry.
4. Explain what DDS and DMD stand for.
5. Identify the eight specialties of dentistry.
6. Describe generally what career skills are performed by dental hygienists, dental assistants, and dental laboratory technicians.
7. List the education required for and the professional organizations that represent each profession.

SUMMARY

It is important to know the historic struggles in and contributions to dentistry that advanced the profession into what it is today. Organized dentistry was formed with the intent to promote the sharing of information concerned with excellence in dentistry. To provide excellence in dentistry, additional dental team members would become recognized and add contributing roles. Therefore, the dental assistant will need to be able to identify and define those who contribute to the dental profession.

KEY TERMS

American Dental Assistants
  Association (ADAA)
American Dental Association (ADA)
American Dental Hygienists'
  Association (ADHA)
American Dental Laboratory
  Technician Association (ADLTA)
certified dental assistant (CDA)

Dental Assisting National Board,
  Inc. (DANB)
dental public health
Dr. C. Edmund Kells
Dr. Greene Vardiman Black
endodontics
forensic dentistry
Juliette Southard

oral and maxillofacial surgery
oral pathology
orthodontics
pediatric dentistry
periodontics
Pierre Fauchard
prosthodontics
Wilhelm Conrad Roentgen

EXERCISES AND ACTIVITIES

1. Dr. Greene Vardiman Black was known as _____
   - A. G.V. Black.
   - B. an inventor of numerous machines for testing alloys.
   - C. an inventor of numerous instruments to refine the cavity prep.
   - D. the "grand old man of dentistry."
   - E. All of the above

2. The ADA represents which professionals? _____
   - A. Hygienists
   - B. Assistants
   - C. Dentists
   - D. Laboratory technicians

3. The ADAA represents which professionals? _____
   - A. Hygienists
   - B. Assistants
   - C. Dentists
   - D. Laboratory technicians

4. An endodontist would handle which of the following? _____
   - A. Oral care in children
   - B. Removal of third molars
   - C. Root canal therapy
   - D. Removal of calculus

5. Orthodontics is the specialty to perform _____
   - A. root canal therapy.
   - B. straightening of the teeth.
   - C. extraction of third molars.
   - D. treatment of surrounding tissues.

6. Pediatric dentistry is the specialty concerned with _____
   - A. geriatric patients.
   - B. extraction of third molars.
   - C. oral care of children.
   - D. straightening teeth with braces.

7. The specialty concerned with the diagnosis and treatment of the diseases of the supporting and surrounding tissues of the tooth is _____
   - A. endodontics.
   - B. orthodontics.
   - C. periodontics.
   - D. pediatric dentistry.

8. The first dentist whose name was recorded, who practiced in 3000 B.C., was _____
   - A. Pierre Fauchard.
   - B. Hesi-Re.
   - C. John Greenwood.
   - D. Guy de Chauliac.

9. Which of the following is NOT considered an auxiliary personnel? _____
   - A. Dental assistant
   - B. Dental hygienist
   - C. Dental lab technician
   - D. Dental receptionist

Match the historian with the contribution.

Historian
10. _____ Hippocrates
11. _____ Guy de Chauliac
12. _____ da Vinci
13. _____ Fauchard
14. _____ Roentgen

Contribution
- A. Discovered x-rays
- B. First to make distinction between premolar and molar
- C. Father of dentistry
- D. Wrote hygienic rules for oral hygiene
- E. Early advocate of treatment of diseased gingival tissue

Oral Health and Nutrition

OBJECTIVES

The student should strive to meet the following objectives and demonstrate an understanding of the facts and principles presented in this chapter:

1. Describe how plaque forms and affects the tooth.
2. Identify motivation tips for oral hygiene for each age group.
3. Identify the oral hygiene aids available to all patients, including manual and automatic.
4. Demonstrate the five toothbrushing techniques.
5. Identify types of dental floss and demonstrate flossing technique.
6. Describe fluoride and its use in dentistry.
7. Define fluoridation and describe its effectiveness on tooth development and the post-eruption stage.
8. List and explain the forms of fluoride. Describe how to prepare a patient and demonstrate fluoride application.
9. Describe how an understanding of nutrition is used in the profession of dental assisting.
10. Define nutrients found in foods, including carbohydrates, fiber, fats, proteins, and amino acids. Explain how they affect oral hygiene.
11. Define a calorie and basal metabolic rate.
12. Identify and explain the function of vitamins, major minerals, and water.

SUMMARY

To be effective in preventive dentistry, the dental assistant must first care for his or her teeth properly and practice good nutrition. Becoming knowledgeable about the oral disease process will aid the dental assistant to educate the public how to prevent it. The dental assistant can then aid patients in maintaining their teeth and gums. In speaking with patients about their home care habits and nutrition, it is important to remember that patients choose their habits for a variety of reasons, including work, student, parent, cultural, religious, or ethical beliefs. The goal of preventive dentistry is that each individual maintain optimal oral health.

KEY TERMS

calories	enamel hypoplasia	malnutrition
caries	essential amino acids	metabolism
demineralization	fluoropatite crystal	mottled enamel
dentifrice	fluoridation	nutrients
diet	fluorosis	plaque
diuretics	halitosis	undernourished
enamel hypocalcification	hydroxyl ion	xerostomia

EXERCISES AND ACTIVITIES

1. Which of the following is NOT a preventative dentistry step for all individuals to follows? _____
   A. Daily brushing and flossing
   B. Good nutrition
   C. Routine dental visits and examination
   D. Sucking on hard candy daily
   E. Occasional use of disclosing agents and evaluation of plaque condition

2. Dental plaque _____
   A. contains bacteria, which grows in colonies.
   B. is a soft, white, sticky mass.
   C. contains bacteria, which is fed by foods we eat.
   D. All of the above

3. Which of the following is the dental decay (caries) equation? _____
   A. Sugar + Protein = Caries + Gingiva = Decay
   B. Sugar + Plaque = Acid + Gingiva = Decay
   C. Sugar + Plaque = Acid + Tooth = Decay
   D. None of the above

4. The use of disclosing agents will _____
   A. replace toothbrushing.
   B. replace flossing.
   C. make plaque visible.
   D. replace the use of dentifrice.

5. What organization awards a Seal of Acceptance classification to products that are safe and effective for self-care? _____
   A. American Dental Hygienists' Association (ADHA)
   B. American Dental Assistants Association (ADAA)
   C. American Dental Association (ADA)
   D. Occupational Health and Safety Administration (OSHA)

6. Mouth rinsing is often used to _____
   A. loosen debris.
   B. temporarily eliminate bad breath.
   C. give patients a pleasant taste.
   D. All of the above.

7. Correct toothbrush design includes _____
   A. bristles that are flexible.
   B. a firm handle.
   C. a lightweight handle.
   D. size and shape for efficient cleaning.
   E. All of the above

8. Dental floss is NOT available in a _____
   A. waxed form.
   B. unwaxed form.
   C. coarse form.
   D. lightly waxed form.
   E. flavored form.

9. How often should the teeth be flossed? _____
   A. Once a week
   B. Daily
   C. Every other day
   D. Every other week

10. A prosthetic device that requires special oral hygiene care is a(n) _____
    A. amalgam.   D. fixed bridge.
    B. composite.   E. third molar.
    C. root canal.

11. Orthodontic appliances must be kept plaque free by using _____
    A. just floss.
    B. soda pop.
    C. apples.
    D. a water irrigation device.

12. Chronic fluoride poisoning can result from _____
    A. ingestion of high fluoride levels in water.
    B. combinations of several fluoride sources over a period of time.
    C. the fluoride level reaching 1.8 ppm to 2.0 ppm
    D. All of the above

13. What is the primary dental health benefit of fluoride? _____
    A. No plaque
    B. Reduction of caries
    C. No calculus
    D. No orthodontics ever needed

14. Fluoride compounds used today are _____
    A. systemic fluoride.
    B. sodium fluoride.
    C. stannous fluoride.
    D. acidulated fluoride.
    E. B, C, D

15. The most important nutrient(s) in the body is (are) _____
    A. water.
    B. vitamins.
    C. minerals.
    D. fluoride.

16. Nutrients are defined as _____
    A. cariogenic food and carbohydrates.
    B. any chemical substance present in food that is necessary for growth.
    C. an undernourished diet.
    D. everything that is taken in the mouth.

17. The number one cause of death of Americans over the age of forty is due to heart disease, and a contributing factor may be the consumption of too many _____
    A. fats.
    B. proteins.
    C. carbohydrates.
    D. foods containing fiber.

18. How many major minerals are found in the body? _____
    A. Ten
    B. Two
    C. Three
    D. Seven

19. The basal metabolic rate (BMR) will NOT be higher for which of the following group of people? _____
    A. Heavier individuals
    B. Pregnant women
    C. Leaner individuals
    D. Developing children

20. Animal proteins, which include _____, are classified complete because they have all ten essential amino acids.
    1. eggs
    2. milk
    3. meat
    4. vegetables
    5. grain protein

    A. 1, 4, 5
    B. 3, 4, 5
    C. 1, 2, 3
    D. 2, 3, 5

21. Which of the following dental aids help to clean between the teeth? _____
    1. Interproximal brush
    2. Rubber stimulator
    3. Wooden stimulator
    4. Dental floss
    5. Water irrigation device
    6. Toothbrush
    7. Disclosing tablet
    8. Chewing gum

    A. 1, 6, 7, 8
    B. 1, 2, 3, 7
    C. 3, 4, 5, 8
    D. 1, 2, 3, 4, 5
    E. 5, 6, 7, 8

Patient motivation is critical for the successful prevention of dental disease. Match the age group with the general characteristics pertaining to that group.

Age Group

22. _____ Infant up to one year
23. _____ Preschool
24. _____ Ages five through eight
25. _____ Ages nine through twelve
26. _____ Ages thirteen through fifteen

General Characteristics

A. Can brush with parent supervision
B. Can brush and begin to floss
C. Oral hygiene performed by parent or caregiver
D. Routinely snacks; rate of decay rising
E. Brushes and flosses proficiently

Following are the various toothbrushing techniques and methods of use. Match the correct toothbrushing technique with its descriptive method.

Brushing Technique

27. _____ Bass or Modified Bass
28. _____ Charters
29. _____ Modified Stillman
30. _____ Rolling Stroke
31. _____ Modified Scrub

Method of Use

A. Activate the brush back and forth (scrubbing motion)
B. Brush is parallel to tooth with bristles pointed apically
C. Removes plaque next to and directly beneath the gingival margin
D. Stimulates gingiva, both the marginal and interdental
E. Bristles of brush are angled against the tooth surface, toward the root

Match the vitamin with how the body uses it.

Vitamin

32. _____ Vitamin A
33. _____ Vitamin D
34. _____ Vitamin K
35. _____ Vitamin C

Use

A. Promotes blood clotting and coagulation
B. Gives strength to epithelial tissue
C. Acts to hold cells together
D. Promotes tooth development

Match the term with the best definition.

Term

36. _____ Fluoride
37. _____ Mottled enamel
38. _____ Optimum level of fluoride
39. _____ Fluoridation
40. _____ Fluoride toxicity

Definition

A. Also known as fluorosis
B. Process of adding fluoride to water supply
C. Essential to formation of healthy bones and teeth
D. Fluoride absorbed in excessive amounts
E. 1 ppm

SKILL COMPETENCY ASSESSMENT

2-1 Applying Disclosing Agent for Plaque Identification

Student's Name _____ Date _____

Instructor's Name _____

SKILL   To identify plaque and its location for patient and operator.

PERFORMANCE OBJECTIVE   The student will demonstrate the application of the disclosing agent.

	Self Evaluation	Student Evaluation	Possible Points	Instructor Evaluation	Comments
Equipment and Supplies					
1. Basic setup: mouth mirror, explorer, cotton pliers			1		
2. Saliva ejector, evacuator tip (HVE), and air-water syringe tip			1		
3. Cotton rolls, cotton-tip applicator, and gauze sponges			1		
4. Petroleum jelly (lubricant)			1		
5. Disclosing agent (liquid or tablet) and dappen dish			1		
6. Plaque chart and red pencil			1		
Competency Steps					
1. The operator examines the oral cavity and reviews the health history.			3		
2. The operator applies the petroleum jelly (lubricant) to the patient's lips (and to any tooth-colored restorations to prevent staining).			2		
3. The operator can apply the liquid using the dappen dish and a cotton-tip applicator. Each attainable surface of the teeth should be covered with the disclosing solution.			2		
4. If using the tablet, the patient chews and swishes around for fifteen seconds.			2		
5. The remaining solution is rinsed and evacuated.			2		
6. The patient uses a hand mirror to see the plaque and the operator uses a mouth mirror and an air-water syringe to identify and chart the plaque.			2		
7. Demonstrate methods of brushing and flossing for plaque removal to the patient.			2		
TOTAL POINTS POSSIBLE			21		
TOTAL POINTS POSSIBLE—2nd Attempt			19		
TOTAL POINTS EARNED			_____		

Points assigned reflect importance of step to meeting objective: Important = 1; Essential = 2; Critical = 3. Students will lose 2 points for repeated attempts. Failure results if any of the critical steps are omitted or performed incorrectly. If using a 100-point scale, determine score by dividing points earned by total points possible and multiplying the results by 100.

SCORE: _____

SKILL COMPETENCY ASSESSMENT

2-2 Bass or Modified Bass Brushing Technique

Student's Name _____ Date _____

Instructor's Name _____

SKILL   To remove plaque next to and directly beneath the gingival margin.

PERFORMANCE OBJECTIVE   The student will demonstrate the application of this toothbrushing technique.

	Self Evaluation	Student Evaluation	Possible Points	Instructor Evaluation	Comments
Equipment and Supplies					
1. Toothbrush			1		
Competency Steps					
1. Grasp the brush and place it so the bristles are at a 45-degree angle, with the tips of the bristles directed straight into the gingival sulcus.			2		
2. Using the tips of the bristles, vibrate back and forth with short, light strokes for a count of 10, allowing the tips of the bristles to enter the sulcus and cover the gingival margin.			3		
3. Lift the brush and continue into the next area or group of teeth until all areas have been cleaned.			1		
4. The toe bristles of the brush can be used to clean the lingual (tongue) anterior area in the arch.			1		

TOTAL POINTS POSSIBLE ———————————————————— 8

TOTAL POINTS POSSIBLE—2nd Attempt   6

TOTAL POINTS EARNED   _____

Points assigned reflect importance of step to meeting objective: Important = 1; Essential = 2; Critical = 3. Students will lose 2 points for repeated attempts. Failure results if any of the critical steps are omitted or performed incorrectly. If using a 100-point scale, determine score by dividing points earned by total points possible and multiplying the results by 100.

SCORE: _____

SKILL COMPETENCY ASSESSMENT

2-3 Dental Flossing Technique *(corresponds to textbook Procedure 2-7)*

Student's Name _____ Date _____

Instructor's Name _____

SKILL To remove the bacterial plaque and other debris from the otherwise inaccessible areas, the proximal surfaces of the teeth.

PERFORMANCE OBJECTIVE The student will demonstrate the application of this flossing technique.

	Self Evaluation	Student Evaluation	Possible Points	Instructor Evaluation	Comments
Equipment and Supplies					
1. Dental floss			1		
Competency Steps					
1. Obtain the appropriate dental floss and dispense.			2		
2. Wrap the ends of the floss around the middle or ring finger as anchors.			3		
3. Grasp the floss between the thumb and index finger of both hands, allowing ½ to 1 inch to remain between the two hands.			2		
4. For the maxillary teeth, pass the floss over the two thumbs and direct the floss upward.			2		
5. For the mandibular teeth, pass the floss over the two index fingers and guide it downward.			2		
6. Direct the floss to pass gently between the teeth, using a sawing motion. Try not to snap the floss through the contacts because it may damage the interdental papilla (gingival point between teeth).			2		
7. Curve the floss in a C-shape to wrap it around the tooth and allow access into the sulcus area. When a resistance is felt, it indicates that the bottom of the gingival sulcus has been reached.			2		
8. Move the floss gently up and down the surface of the tooth to remove the plaque.			2		
9. Lift slightly and wrap the floss in the opposite direction in a C-shape over the adjacent tooth.			2		
10. Move the floss gently up and down the surface of this tooth prior to removing it from the area.			2		
11. Rotate the floss on the fingers to allow for a fresh section to be used each time, and continue to clean between each and every tooth. Be systematic so no areas are missed.			1		
12. Use the dental floss around the distal surface of the most posterior tooth by wrapping it in a tight C-shape and moving it gently up and down with a firm pressure.			1		

2-3 continued

	Self Evaluation	Student Evaluation	Possible Points	Instructor Evaluation	Comments
13. Do the most posterior teeth in all four quadrants in the same manner.			1		

TOTAL POINTS POSSIBLE   25

TOTAL POINTS POSSIBLE—2nd Attempt   23

TOTAL POINTS EARNED   _____

Points assigned reflect importance of step to meeting objective: Important = 1; Essential = 2; Critical = 3. Students will lose 2 points for repeated attempts. Failure results if any of the critical steps are omitted or performed incorrectly. If using a 100-point scale, determine score by dividing points earned by total points possible and multiplying the results by 100.

SCORE: _____

SKILL COMPETENCY ASSESSMENT

2-4 Fluoride Application *(corresponds to textbook Procedure 2-8)*

Student's Name _____ Date _____

Instructor's Name _____

SKILL   To apply topical fluoride after either toothbrushing or a rubber-cup polish. Fluoride penetrates only the outer layer of the enamel if the tooth is clean.

PERFORMANCE OBJECTIVE   The student will demonstrate the application of this topical fluoride technique.

	Self Evaluation	Student Evaluation	Possible Points	Instructor Evaluation	Comments
Equipment and Supplies					
1. Basic setup: mouth mirror, explorer, and cotton pliers			1		
2. Saliva ejector, evacuator tip (HVE), air-water tip			1		
3. Cotton rolls, gauze sponges			1		
4. Fluoride solution			1		
5. Appropriately sized trays			1		
6. Timer (for one or four minutes)			1		
Competency Steps					
1. Seat the patient in an upright position, review health history, and confirm he or she has not had allergic reactions to fluorides.			2		
2. Explain the procedure to the patient. Inform the patient to try to not swallow the fluoride and show him or her how to use the saliva ejector.			3		
3. Explain to the patient that for the fluoride to be most effective, he or she should not eat, drink, or rinse for thirty minutes after the fluoride treatment.			2		
4. Select the trays and try them in the patient's mouth to ensure coverage of all the exposed teeth.			2		
5. Place the fluoride gel or foam in the tray. The tray should be about one-third full.			2		
6. Dry all the teeth with the air syringe. To keep the teeth dry while reaching for the tray, keep your finger in the patient's mouth and tell the patient to keep it open.			2		
7. Place the tray over the dried teeth. The maxillary and mandibular arches can be done at the same time or individually.			2		
8. Move the trays up and down to dispense the fluoride solution around the teeth.			2		

2-4 continued

	Self Evaluation	Student Evaluation	Possible Points	Instructor Evaluation	Comments
9. Place the saliva ejector between the arches and have the patient close gently.			2		
10. Set the timer for the designated amount of time.			2		
11. When the timer goes off, remove the saliva ejector and the trays from the patient's mouth.			1		
12. Quickly evacuate the mouth with the saliva ejector or the evacuator (HVE) completely to remove any excess fluid.			1		
13. Remind the patient not to eat, drink, or rinse for thirty minutes.			1		
14. Make the chart entry, including the date, the fluoride solution applied, and any reactions.			1		

TOTAL POINTS POSSIBLE   31

TOTAL POINTS POSSIBLE—2nd Attempt   29

TOTAL POINTS EARNED   _____

Points assigned reflect importance of step to meeting objective: Important = 1; Essential = 2; Critical = 3. Students will lose 2 points for repeated attempts. Failure results if any of the critical steps are omitted or performed incorrectly. If using a 100-point scale, determine score by dividing points earned by total points possible and multiplying the results by 100.

SCORE: _____

General Anatomy and Physiology

OBJECTIVES

The student should strive to meet the following objectives and demonstrate an understanding of the facts and principles presented in this chapter:

1. List the body systems, body planes and directions, and cavities of the body, and describe the structure and function of the cell.
2. Explain the functions and divisions of the skeletal system, list the composition of the bone, and identify the types of joints.
3. List the functions and parts of the muscular system.
4. List the functions and the structure of the nervous system.
5. List the functions and the parts of the endocrine system.
6. Explain the dental concerns related to the reproductive system.
7. Explain the functions of the circulatory system and list and identify the parts.
8. Explain the functions and parts of the digestive system.
9. List the functions and parts of the respiratory system.
10. List the functions and parts of the lymphatic system and the immune system.

SUMMARY

Specific terms are used to establish a means for the health professional to communicate more effectively. Depending on the information and understanding needed, the human body can be studied on many different levels. The body is divided into systems, planes, cavities, and basic units. This gives common references and terms for studying and communicating information about the human body.

The dental assistant needs to be familiar with the terminology of body systems and how each system functions to give the quality of care each patient deserves. An understanding of both the anatomy and physiology of each body system is needed.

KEY TERMS

absorption process	chyme	myocardium
alimentary canal	dorsal cavity	nasopharynx
alveoli	endocardium	oropharynx
articulations	epiglottis	osteoblasts
atria	hemostasis	osteoclast
bronchioles	homeostasis	pericardium
cancellous bone	laryngopharynx	periosteum
cartilage	myelin sheath	ventral cavity

EXERCISES AND ACTIVITIES

1. _____ is the study of the body structure.
   - A. Physiology
   - B. Anatomy
   - C. Alimentary
   - D. Articulation

2. _____ is the study of the body functions.
   - A. Anatomy
   - B. Physiology
   - C. Pericardium
   - D. Periosteum

3. Which of the following is not a system of the body? _____
   - A. Skeletal
   - B. Anterior
   - C. Muscle
   - D. Nerves
   - E. Endocrine

4. _____ refers to the front of the body or body section.
   - A. Dorsal
   - B. Inferior
   - C. Medial
   - D. Anterior

5. _____ refers to the back of the body or body section.
   - A. Proximal
   - B. Anterior
   - C. Posterior
   - D. Mesial

6. _____ means toward the midline of the body.
   - A. Proximal
   - B. Mesial
   - C. Distal
   - D. Lateral

7. _____ refers to the part of the body closest to the point of attachment.
   - A. Inferior
   - B. Superior
   - C. Dorsal
   - D. Proximal
   - E. Posterior

8. Which of the following planes divides the body into left and right halves? _____
   - A. Frontal
   - B. Transverse
   - C. Horizontal
   - D. Sagittal

9. Which of the following planes divides the body into front and back sections? _____
   - A. Transverse
   - B. Frontal
   - C. Mid-sagittal
   - D. Sagittal

10. The dorsal cavity shares one continuous space with the spinal canal and the _____
    - A. thoracic cavity.
    - B. abdominal cavity.
    - C. pelvic cavity.
    - D. digestive tract.
    - E. cranial cavity.

11. The basic unit of all systems and the smallest functioning unit of the body is called _____
    - A. cell.
    - B. tissue.
    - C. organ.
    - D. muscle.

12. The axial skeleton includes the _____
    - A. bones of the cranium.
    - B. bones of the face.
    - C. spinal column.
    - D. ribs.
    - E. All of the above

13. In an adult skeleton, there are _____ bones.
    - A. 300
    - B. 200
    - C. 216
    - D. 206

14. The periosteum contains _____
    - A. blood vessels.
    - B. lymph vessels.
    - C. osteoblasts.
    - D. nerve tissue.
    - E. All of the above

15. _____ marrow contains mainly fat cells.
    - A. Red
    - B. Yellow
    - C. White
    - D. Clear

16. _____ bones support the teeth and surrounding tissues.
    - A. Synovial
    - B. Facial
    - C. Osteoclastic
    - D. Cartilaginous

17. A condition or disease of the skeletal system is _____
    - A. indigestion.
    - B. fibromyalgia.
    - C. homeostasis.
    - D. osteoporosis.

18. The loss of bony material, leaving bone brittle is _____
    - A. osteomyelitis.
    - B. periosteum.
    - C. osteoblasts.
    - D. osteoporosis.

19. The _____ muscle will move food along the digestive track and keeps the heart beating.
    - A. internal
    - B. external
    - C. posterior
    - D. anterior

20. What muscle type has the largest amount of muscle tissue? _____
    - A. Cardiac
    - B. Striated
    - C. Non-striated
    - D. Fascia

21. When muscles contract they become _____
    A. shorter.   C. A, B
    B. thicker.   D. None of the above

22. _____ are composed of bands or sheets of fibrous tissue and act to connect or support two or more bones.
    A. Fibers   C. Tendons
    B. Ligaments   D. Joints

23. The _____ point of the muscle is where the bone is movable.
    A. isotonic   C. isometric
    B. aponeurosis   D. insertion

24. When assisting with dental procedures, dental assistants use their back and neck, putting stress and strain on the _____ system.
    A. reproductive   C. endocrine
    B. muscular   D. respiratory

25. If muscles are not used, they begin to deteriorate. This condition is known as _____
    A. atrophy.   C. spasticity.
    B. fibromyalgia.   D. gravis.

26. The specialized group of peripheral nerves that function mainly automatically are called _____
    A. PMS.   C. CNS.
    B. PNS.   D. ANS.

27. The nerve fibers that conduct impulses to the cell body are called _____
    A. axons.   C. synapses.
    B. dendrites.   D. myelin.

28. Which of the following statements is not true of the spinal cord? _____
    A. It is part of the reproductive system.
    B. It is a center for reflex responses.
    C. It generally protects the body from stressful situations.
    D. It transmits stimuli from the body to the brain.

29. The cranial nerves that are related directly to the oral cavity are the _____
    A. fourth and seventh.
    B. seventh and twelfth.
    C. second and fifth.
    D. fifth and seventh.

30. What system is affected when the patient is administered a pain blocker? _____
    A. Skeletal   C. Muscular
    B. Nervous   D. Respiratory

31. _____ is a sudden onset of facial paralysis.
    A. Multiple sclerosis
    B. Parkinson's disease
    C. Neuritis
    D. Bell's palsy

32. The endocrine system generally controls _____
    A. the production of insulin.
    B. the breakdown of glycogen.
    C. the impulses of muscles.
    D. circulatory congestion in bone marrow.

33. Major glands of the endocrine system include _____
    A. respiratory.   D. muscular.
    B. adrenal.   E. reproductive.
    C. neuritis.

34. The condition in which the thyroid gland is underactive is called _____
    A. hypothyroidism.   C. pericardium.
    B. hyperthyroidism. D. myocardium.

35. The pathway that carries the blood from the aorta to the smallest blood vessels back to the heart is called _____ circulation.
    A. pulmonary   C. pericardium
    B. systemic   D. myocardium

36. The thin lining on the inside of the heart is called the _____
    A. pericardium.   C. endocardium.
    B. myocardium.   D. atrium.

37. _____ carry oxygenated blood from the heart to the capillaries.
    A. Veins   C. Arterioles
    B. Capillaries   D. Arteries

38. _____ carry blood drained from capillaries back to the heart.
    A. Veins   C. Arterioles
    B. Capillaries   D. Arteries

39. The _____ are the connection between the arteries and the veins.
    A. veins   C. arterioles
    B. capillaries   D. arteries

40. What is the liquid portion of the blood called? _____
    A. Plasma   C. Capillaries
    B. Arteries   D. Veins

41. What are the cells or solid portion of the blood called? _____
    A. Blood   C. Capillaries
    B. Plasma   D. Corpuscles

42. Red blood cells contain the protein called _____
    A. leukemia.   C. hemostasis.
    B. thrombocytes. D. hemoglobin.

43. A disorder called _____ is the failure of the blood to clot.
    A. hypothyroidism   C. leukemia
    B. hyperthyroidism D. hemophilia

44. The alimentary canal does not include the _____
    A. pharynx.   C. stomach.
    B. esophagus.   D. atrium.

Head and Neck Anatomy

The student should strive to meet the following objectives and demonstrate an understanding of the facts and principles presented in this chapter:

1. List and identify the landmarks of the face and the oral cavity.
2. Identify the bones of the cranium and the face and identify the landmarks on the maxilla and the mandible.
3. List and identify the muscles of mastication, facial expression, the floor of the mouth, the tongue, the throat, the neck, and the shoulders. Explain their functions.
4. List and identify the nerves of the maxilla and the mandible.
5. Identify the arteries and veins of the head and the neck.

SUMMARY

As a vital team member, the dental assistant needs to be able to recognize factors that may influence the general physical health of the patient. The understanding of landmarks of the oral cavity, as well as being able to describe head and neck anatomy as it relates to location of structure and function, will enable the dental assistant to recognize the abnormal. For this reason, accuracy is especially important when completing the patient's dental chart. This information will provide a point of comparison for future visits.

KEY TERMS

alveolar process
buccal branch
buccinator
common carotid
ethmoid bone
external jugular vein
external oblique ridge
external pterygoid muscles
frena
incisive nerve branch
incisive papilla

inferior alveolar branch
internal jugular vein
internal oblique ridge
internal pterygoid muscles
labial commissures
labio-mental groove
lacrimal bones
linea alba
lingual branch
masseter muscles
mental nerve branch

mentalis
oral vestibule
papilla
parotid glands
sphenoid bone
Stensen's duct
temporal muscles
uvula
vermilion border
Wharton's duct
zygomatic bones

EXERCISES AND ACTIVITIES

1. The lips are covered externally with _____
    A. skin.
    B. mucous membranes.
    C. lingual mucosa.
    D. gingival papilla.

2. The outer edge of the nostril is referred to as the _____
    1. groove.
    2. wing.
    3. shallow, V-shaped depression.
    4. ala of the nose.
    5. philtrum.

    A. 1, 2, 5
    B. 2, 4, 5
    C. 1, 3, 5
    D. 2, 4
    E. 3, 4, 5

3. The portion of the lips called the labial commissures is examined for _____
    A. cracks.
    B. color change.
    C. variations in form.
    D. All of the above

Using the diagram below, identify the landmarks with the correct term.

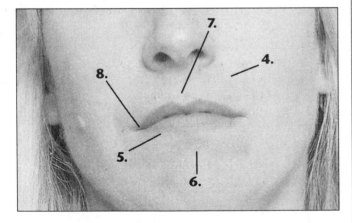

4. _____
5. _____
6. _____
7. _____
8. _____

A. Labial commissure
B. Labio-mental groove
C. Naso-labial groove
D. Philtrum
E. Vermilion border

9. Which of the following landmarks is not a part of the oral cavity? _____
    A. Vestibule   D. Gingiva
    B. Lips   E. Frenum
    C. Stensen's duct

10. The deepest part of the oral vestibule is called the _____
    A. fornix U shape.
    B. philtrum V shape.
    C. vermilion.
    D. commissures.

11. The tissue that lines the inner surface of the lips and cheeks is called _____
    A. papilla.   C. frenum.
    B. gingiva.   D. mucosa.

12. On the labial mucosa are yellowish glands just inside the commissures called _____
    A. Fordyce's spots.   C. linea alba.
    B. fornix.   D. uvula.

13. On the buccal mucosa is a raised white line that runs parallel to where the teeth meet, called the _____
    A. vestibule.   C. fornix.
    B. frenum.   D. linea alba.

14. The main frena of the maxillary are between the _____
    A. premolars.   C. laterals.
    B. centrals.   D. third molars.

15. The inside palate area of the maxillary teeth is often referred to as the _____
    A. sulcus.
    B. roof of the mouth.
    C. filiform.
    D. duct.

16. The occasional lump or prominence of bone in the maxillary palate is called a _____
    A. torus.   C. fauces.
    B. uvula.   D. frenum.

17. The projection that extends off the back of the maxillary soft palate is the _____
    A. frenum.   C. papilla.
    B. uvula.   D. commissures.

18. Covering the dorsal side of the tongue are small raised projections called _____, where taste buds are located.
    A. foliate   C. sulcus
    B. papilla   D. fauces

19. Covering the dorsal of the tongue are hair-like projections called _____
    A. circumvallate papillae.
    B. filiform papillae.
    C. fungiform papillae.
    D. foliate papillae.

20. Name the sulcus that marks the end of the alveolar ridge and the beginning of the floor of the mouth. _____
    A. Sublingual caruncles
    B. Sublingual folds
    C. Sublingual sulcus
    D. Sublingual gland

21. The largest of the salivary glands are the _____
    A. parotid.   C. subcaruncles.
    B. submandibular.   D. sublingual.

22. The Wharton's duct empties saliva from which gland? _____
    A. Parotid   C. Submandibular
    B. Fauces   D. Terminalis

23. The mumps are a viral infection affecting which gland? _____
    A. Salivary   C. Submandibular
    B. Parotid   D. Wharton's

24. The bone that contains the mastoid process is the _____
    A. parietal.   C. frontal.
    B. temporal.   D. occipital.

25. Which bone forms part of the nose, orbits, and the floor of the cranium? _____
    A. Sphenoid   C. Pterygoid
    B. Ethmoid   D. Styloid

26. The _____ bone is one continuous bone that goes across the skull anterior to the temporal bones and is shaped like a bat with its wings spread out.
    A. styloid   C. sphenoid
    B. occipital   D. pterygoid

27. What bone forms the cheeks?
    A. Vomer   C. Lacrimal
    B. Nasal   D. Zygomatic

28. The tear ducts pass through which bones? _____
    A. Zygomatic   C. Vomer
    B. Nasal   D. Lacrimal

29. The largest of the facial bones, which is composed of two sections, is the _____
    A. maxilla.   C. palatine.
    B. mandible.   D. rami.

30. The only movable bone of the face is the _____
    A. maxilla.   C. rami.
    B. mandible.   D. palatine.

31. The _____ process forms the bone that supports the maxillary teeth.
    A. alveolar   C. zygomatic
    B. palatine   D. median

32. The _____ articulates with the temporal bones to form the temporomandibular joint.
    A. palatine   C. foramen
    B. condyle   D. symphysis

33. The temporal muscles of mastication function to _____
    A. depress the mandible.
    B. depress the maxilla.
    C. expand the posterior fibers.
    D. elevate the mandible.

34. The masseter muscles belong to which group of muscles of the head and neck? _____
    A. Muscles of facial expression
    B. Muscles of the floor of the mouth
    C. Muscles of the tongue
    D. Muscles of mastication

35. This muscle is the medial surface of the lateral pterygoid plate, otherwise known as _____
    A. external pterygoid.
    B. internal pterygoid.
    C. temporals.
    D. masseter.

36. The buccinator muscle belongs to which of the following groups? _____
    A. Muscles of facial expression
    B. Muscles of the floor of the mouth
    C. Muscles of the tongue
    D. Muscles of mastication

37. The function of this muscle is to wrinkle the skin of the chin. _____
    A. Buccinator   C. Orbicularis
    B. Oris   D. Mentalis

38. One of the muscles that serves to form the floor of the mouth is the _____
    A. digastric. C. hypoglossus.
    B. genioglossus. D. styloglossus.

39. The largest cranial nerve, which innervates the maxilla and the mandible, is the _____
    A. ophthalmic. C. nasopalatine.
    B. trigeminal. D. infraorbital.

40. What nerve branch is composed of both sensory and motor nerves? _____
    A. Lingual C. Buccal
    B. Inferior alveolar D. Mandibular

41. The buccal nerve branch innervates which of the following? _____
    1. Lingual mucosa
    2. Buccal mucosa
    3. Posterior alveolar
    4. Buccal gingiva
    5. Buccal of the mandibular molars
    6. Mylohyoid

    A. 1, 3
    B. 2, 3, 4
    C. 2, 4, 6
    D. 2, 4, 5

42. The external jugular vein _____
    A. receives blood from the cranium.
    B. receives blood from the face.
    C. receives blood from the neck.
    D. drains blood from the superficial veins of the face and neck.

43. The internal jugular vein _____
    A. receives blood from the cranium.
    B. drains blood from the superficial veins of the face and neck.
    C. drains blood from the neck.
    D. drains blood from the cranium.

Match the following landmarks with the correct description.

Landmark
44. _____ Palate
45. _____ Incisive papilla
46. _____ Palatine raphe
47. _____ Palatine rugae
48. _____ Torus

Description
A. Prominence of bone in middle maxillary palate
B. Raised line posterior, middle of hard palate
C. Ridges that run horizontal across hard palate
D. Raised area of tissue behind maxillary central incisors
E. Roof of the mouth

These nerve branches descend from the mandibular nerve. Match the nerve branch with its service.

Nerve Branch
49. _____ Lingual
50. _____ Inferior alveolar
51. _____ Mental
52. _____ Incisive

Service
A. Runs parallel to lingual nerve
B. Supplies chin and lower lip area
C. Innervates anterior teeth and labial gingiva
D. Descends to the underside of tongue

Embryology and Histology

OBJECTIVES

The student should strive to meet the following objectives and demonstrate an understanding of the facts and principles presented in this chapter:

1. Identify the terms and times of the three prenatal phases of pregnancy.
2. Describe how the human face develops and changes during the zygote and embryo phases.
3. Describe the life cycle of a tooth and identify the stages.
4. Identify the four primary structures of the tooth and the location and function of each.
5. Identify the substances of enamel, dentin, cementum, and pulp and their identifying marks.
6. Identify the components of the periodontium and the considerations of the aveolar bone.
7. Describe the structures of the gingiva and the mucosa.

SUMMARY

It is vital for the entire dental team to be able to communicate the structure and function of the oral cavity. Therefore, it is important for the dental assistant to understand the structure/function of tissue, the prenatal growth/development process of oral embryology, and the oral cavity that surrounds the teeth.

KEY TERMS

alveolar crest
alveolar mucosa
alveolar process
alveolus
ameloblasts
attached gingiva
attrition
calcification
cementoblasts
cementum
cleft lip

cleft palate
cleft uvula
dentin
dentinal tubules
enamel
epithelial attachment
fibroblasts
free gingiva
gingiva
gingival sulcus

lamina dura
mucogingival junction
Nasmyth's membrane
odontoblasts
periodontium
philtrum
pulp
Sharpey's fibers
stomedeum
zygote

EXERCISES AND ACTIVITIES

1. _____ is the study of prenatal growth and development of an individual.
   - A. Histology
   - B. Microbiology
   - C. Physiology
   - D. Embryology

2. What are three primary embryonic layers formed early in the embryo phase? _____
   1. Ectoderm
   2. Mesoderm
   3. Proliferate
   4. Philtrum
   5. Endoderm
   6. Stomedeum

   - A. 1, 2, 5
   - B. 2, 5, 6
   - C. 1, 2, 3
   - D. 1, 2, 4

3. During the _____ phase, the development of different tissues takes place.
   - A. morphodifferentiation
   - B. cytodifferentiation
   - C. histodifferentiation
   - D. nasolacrimal

4. In which week of the prenatal development will the face begin to form? _____
   - A. Twelfth
   - B. Fourth
   - C. Sixteenth
   - D. Ninth

5. In the facial development phase, what stage is responsible for forming the upper portion of the face, forehead, eyes, and nose? _____
   - A. Medial nasal
   - B. Mandibular process
   - C. Frontonasal process
   - D. Stomedeum

6. In the facial development phase, what stage is responsible for forming the cheeks, sides of the upper lip, and maxilla? _____
   - A. Medial nasal
   - B. Mandibular process
   - C. Frontonasal process
   - D. Stomedeum

7. What factors can initiate malformation in the unborn child? _____
   - A. Genetics
   - B. Environment
   - C. Drugs
   - D. Infections
   - E. All of the above

8. FAS symptoms in an infant are a result of the mother _____
   - A. contracting infections.
   - B. persisting in taking alcohol.
   - C. contracting syphilis.
   - D. being exposed to measles.

9. If a cleft lip occurs on both sides of the lip, it is called _____
   - A. unilateral.
   - B. bilateral.

10. The first stage of the life cycle of the tooth is called _____
    - A. initiation.
    - B. lamina.
    - C. odontogenesis.
    - D. proliferation.

The life cycle of a tooth will go through various development stages. Match the cycle with its proper stage.

Cycle

11. _____ Initiation
12. _____ Proliferation
13. _____ Hisodifferentiation
14. _____ Apposition

Stage

A. Bell
B. Cap
C. Maturation
D. Bud

15. Enamel-forming cells are called _____
    - A. odontoblasts.
    - B. cementoblasts.
    - C. ameloblasts.
    - D. buds.

16. The last development stage prior to eruption is _____
    - A. eruption.
    - B. calcification.
    - C. attrition.
    - D. proliferation.

17. The final stage of the life cycle of the tooth is _____
    - A. initiation.
    - B. proliferation.
    - C. calcification.
    - D. eruption.
    - E. attrition.

18. The study of microscopic structure and function of tissues is _____
    - A. physiology.
    - B. histology.
    - C. embryology.
    - D. microbiology.

19. The hardest living tissue in the body is _____
    - A. dentin.
    - B. cementum.
    - C. enamel.
    - D. lamina.

Match the tooth structure with its description.

Structure
20. _____ Dentin
21. _____ Cementum
22. _____ Pulp tissue
23. _____ Pulp canal
24. _____ Pulp chamber

Description
A. Located in roots of teeth
B. A large portion of the pulp, which is located in crown of tooth
C. Not visible but makes up bulk of tooth structure
D. Located around root; covers the dentin on root portion
E. Located at center of tooth; made up of nerves, blood vessels

25. Primary teeth may erupt with a covering over the enamel, called _____
   A. lines of Retzius.
   B. Tome's process.
   C. perikymata.
   D. Nasmyth's membrane.

26. Which of the following is less hard than enamel but harder than cementum and bone? _____
   A. Dentin   C. Osteoblast
   B. Fibroblast   D. Osteoclast

27. _____ tubules pass through the entire surface of the dentin.
   A. Tertiary   C. Circumpulpal
   B. Mantle   D. Dentinal

28. The most pronounced stained contour line, which occurs due to the trauma of birth, is _____
   A. imbrication.   C. apposition.
   B. contour.   D. neonatal.

Dentin will differ from area to area and is not uniform throughout. Identify the types of dentin and their functions.

Types of Dentin
29. _____ Intertubular
30. _____ Circumpulpal
31. _____ Primary
32. _____ Secondary
33. _____ Tertiary

Function
A. Repairs and is reactive to irritations
B. Forms after completion of apical foramen
C. Found between the tubules
D. Forms the bulk of the tooth
E. Layer of dentin that surrounds pulp

34. Which of the following are functions of pulp? _____
   1. To provide nourishment
   2. To support the dentin
   3. To provide maintenance for the dentin
   4. To transmit sensory information to brain
   5. To identify temperature changes
   6. To identify chemical changes
   7. To pick up plaque easily
   8. To provide mineralization

   A. 1, 7, 8
   B. 1, 2, 3, 4, 5, 6
   C. 1, 2, 3, 7
   D. 3, 4, 6, 8

35. The pulp is partially made from _____, cells from which connective tissue evolves.
   A. pulpitis   C. collagen
   B. dentinal   D. fibroblasts

36. If the pulp is damaged due to an injury, the tissue may become inflamed, causing _____
   A. dentinal hypersensitivity.
   B. pulpitis.
   C. dysplasia.
   D. fibroblasts.

37. The _____ consists of portions of the tooth structure, supporting hard and soft dental tissues, and the alveolar bone.
   A. enamel   C. periodontium
   B. dentin   D. cementum

38. Which of the following are characteristics of cementum? _____
    1. Supports soft dental tissues
    2. Will regenerate like bone
    3. Lighter than dentin
    4. Darker than enamel
    5. Dull light pink in color
    6. Harder than dentin

    A. 1, 3
    B. 2, 4
    C. 3, 4
    D. 1, 4

39. The collagen fibers that act as anchors between the alveolar bone and teeth are referred to as _____
    A. lines of Owen.
    B. lines of Von Ebner.
    C. Sharpey's fibers.
    D. Tome's process.

40. The bones of the mandible and maxilla are formed by _____
    A. osteoblasts.   C. alveolus.
    B. osteoclasts.   D. lamina.

41. The cells that remodel and resorb bone are called _____
    A. osteoblasts.   C. alveolus.
    B. osteoclasts.   D. lamina.

42. The extended areas of bone in each arch that are tooth bearing are called the _____
    A. alveolar crest.
    B. alveolus.
    C. alveolar process.
    D. lamina dura.

43. Two cortical bone plates come together between each tooth. This is referred to as the _____
    A. alveolar crest.
    B. alveolus.
    C. alveolar process.
    D. lamina dura.

44. On a dental radiograph, the radiopaque line, or _____ _____, represents the thin, compact alveolus bone lining the socket.
    A. alveolar crest
    B. periodontal ligament
    C. alveolar process
    D. lamina dura

45. The periodontal ligament, like all connective tissue, is formed by _____ cells.
    A. odontoblast   C. osteoblast
    B. fibroblast   D. osteoclast

46. _____ mucosa flows into the tissue of the cheeks, lips, and inside floor of the mandible.
    A. Circular   C. Oblique
    B. Alveolar   D. Apical

47. Which of the following are characteristics of healthy gingiva? _____
    1. Firm tissue surrounding teeth
    2. Stippled texture
    3. Can be attached to underlying bone
    4. Surrounds the root
    5. Thicker at root
    6. Mass attached to dentin

    A. 1, 3, 5
    B. 2, 3, 5
    C. 3, 4, 5
    D. 1, 2, 3

48. Free gingiva is also known as _____
    A. interdental.   C. attached.
    B. epithelial.   D. marginal.

49. The mucogingival junction is the line of demarcation between the _____ gingiva and _____ mucosa.
    A. free, dentinal
    B. attached, alveolar
    C. interdental, alveolar
    D. sulcus, dentinal

50. The space between the unattached gingiva and the tooth is the _____ _____
    A. attached gingiva.
    B. marginal gingiva.
    C. interdental gingiva.
    D. gingival sulcus.

51. In the floor of the gingival sulcus, the _____ attachment attaches to the enamel surface of the teeth.
    A. attached   C. interdental
    B. marginal   D. epithelial

52. In a healthy mouth, the gingival sulcus space would not exceed _____ in depth.
    A. two to three millimeters
    B. three to four millimeters
    C. four to five millimeters
    D. two to four millimeters

There are three prenatal phases of pregnancy. Match the terms with the times.

Terms

53. _____ Zygote
54. _____ Embryo
55. _____ Fetus

Times

A. Two weeks through the eighth week
B. Nine weeks through birth
C. Conception through the first two weeks

Following is a way to remember the primary embryonic layers:

Terms

56. _____ Derm
57. _____ Ecto
58. _____ Meso
59. _____ Endo

Definition

A. Outside
B. Inside
C. Tissue
D. Middle

Tooth Morphology

OBJECTIVES

The student should strive to meet the following objectives and demonstrate an understanding of the facts and principles presented in this chapter:

1. Identify the dental arches and quadrants using the correct terminology.
2. List the primary and permanent teeth by name and location.
3. Explain the eruption schedule for the primary and permanent teeth.
4. Identify the different divisions of the tooth, including clinical and anatomical divisions.
5. Identify the surfaces of each tooth and their locations.
6. List the anatomical structures and their definitions.
7. Describe each permanent tooth according to location, anatomical features, morphology, function, position, and other identifying factors.
8. Describe each deciduous (primary) tooth according to its location, anatomical features, morphology, function, position, and other identifying factors.

SUMMARY

By understanding tooth morphology, the assistant will be better prepared to record accurately for the dentist or hygienist and will make a vital contribution to those individuals to make a more accurate diagnosis. Therefore, the dental assistant will need to be able to identify each tooth form from its anatomical form.

KEY TERMS

adjacent
anatomical crown
apical foramen
bifurcated
buccal
cervical line
cingulum
clinical crown
cusp of Carabelli
cusps
dentition
developmental groove
distal

facial
fissure
fossa
furcation
imbrication lines
incisal edge
lingual
lobes
mamelons
mandibular arch
marginal ridge
maxillary arch

mesial
midline
oblique ridge
occlusal
pit
posterior
ridge
succedaneous
supplemental groove
transverse ridge
triangular ridge
trifurcated

EXERCISES AND ACTIVITIES

Identification of key surfaces of teeth

1. The surface that is toward the midline is called _____
   A. labial.   C. mesial.
   B. distal.   D. lingual.

2. The surface that is away from the midline is called _____
   A. lingual.   C. mesial.
   B. distal.   D. facial.

3. The anatomical crown portion of the tooth is covered with _____
   A. dentin.   C. enamel.
   B. cementum.   D. fiber.

4. The anatomical root is the portion of the tooth covered with _____
   A. enamel.   C. apex.
   B. cementrum.   D. mamelons.

5. The primary (deciduous) dentition consists of _____
   A. thirty-two teeth, eighteen in each arch, nine in each quadrant.
   B. twenty teeth, ten in each arch, five in each quadrant.
   C. sixteen teeth, eight in each arch, four in each quadrant.
   D. twelve teeth, six in each arch, three in each quadrant.

Match each term with its proper definition.

Term

6. _____ Midline
7. _____ Quadrant
8. _____ Maxillary
9. _____ Mandibular

Definition
A. Upper arch
B. Division between two equal halves
C. Lower arch
D. One-fourth of the complete dentition

10. The primary first molar is replaced by an adult _____
    A. canine.   C. first molar.
    B. premolar.   D. lateral.

11. The only permanent teeth that are not succedaneous teeth are the _____
    A. laterals.   C. premolars.
    B. canines.   D. molars.

Match the following terms with the deciduous teeth in the diagram below.

A. Canine
B. Central incisor
C. First molar
D. Second molar
E. Lateral

12. _____
13. _____
14. _____
15. _____
16. _____

Dental Charting

OBJECTIVES

The student should strive to meet the following objectives and demonstrate an understanding of the facts and principles presented in this chapter:

1. Explain why charting is used in most dental practices.
2. Identify charts that use symbols to represent conditions present in the oral cavity.
3. List and explain the systems used for charting the permanent and deciduous dentitions.
4. Define G.V. Black's six classifications of cavity preparations.
5. List common abbreviations used to identify simple, compound, and complex cavities.
6. Describe basic terminology used in dental charting.
7. Explain color indicators and identify charting symbols.

SUMMARY

Dental charting provides legal documentation of the patient's oral cavity. Utilizing the correct numbering system and charting symbols will ensure proper documentation. Therefore, accuracy in charting is critical.

KEY TERMS

abscess
bridge
crown
denture
drifting
Fédération Dentaire Internationale (FDI) system for numbering

gold foil
incipient
mobility
overhang
Palmer System for numbering
partial denture

periodontal pocket
restoration
root canal
sealant
Universal/National System for numbering

EXERCISES AND ACTIVITIES

1. _____ dentistry uses patients' dental records to identify individuals involved in tragedies.
   A. Pediatric
   C. Prosthodontic
   B. Orthodontic
   D. Forensic

2. Most dental charts will show _____
   1. anatomic representation of teeth.
   2. geometric representation of teeth.
   3. cavity classification.
   4. primary dentition.
   5. abbreviated tooth surfaces.
   6. permanent dentition.

   A. 1, 2, 3, 5
   B. 1, 2, 4, 6
   C. 1, 2, 3, 4
   D. 2, 3, 4, 6

3. _____ is the most common numbering system in the United States.
   A. Universal/National System
   B. Fédération Dentaire Internationale System
   C. International Standards Organization
   D. Palmer System

4. How many original standard classifications of cavities were first developed by G.V. Black? _____
   A. One
   D. Four
   B. Two
   E. Five
   C. Three

5. A _____ cavity involves the incisal and/or an occlusal surface worn away due to abrasion.
   A. Class I
   D. Class VI
   B. Class II
   E. Class V
   C. Class IV

6. Which of the following cavities would be referred to as simple? _____
   1. Class I
   2. Class II
   3. Class III
   4. Class V
   5. Class VI
   6. Class IV

   A. 1, 2, 5
   B. 1, 4, 5
   C. 1, 3, 4
   D. 2, 3, 6

7. What would the abbreviation notation be for mesio-occluso-disto-bucco-lingual? _____
   A. MODL
   C. MODBL
   B. MIDB
   D. MDOI

8. The attaching sides of a bridge are called _____
   A. pontics.
   C. cantilevers.
   B. plates.
   D. abutments.

9. The portion of a bridge that replaces the missing tooth is called a(n) _____
   A. abutment.
   C. plate.
   B. pontic.
   D. denture.

10. _____ is a term used to identify a localized area of infection.
    A. Incipient
    C. Sealant
    B. Decay
    D. Abscess

11. All teeth support each other. _____ can occur when a tooth is removed and a space is created.
    A. Drifting
    C. Periodontal disease
    B. Overhang
    D. Abscess

12. _____ refers to an area that does not yet show decay, but the surface has begun to decalcify.
    A. Gold foil
    C. Sealant
    B. Incipient
    D. Cavity

13. _____ is the result of excessive restorative material.
    A. Pocket
    C. Sealant
    B. Overhang
    D. Root canal

14. What prosthetic device replaces missing teeth by metal framework and artificial teeth? _____
    A. Upper plate
    B. Full denture
    C. Partial denture
    D. Bridge
    E. Maryland bridge

15. _____ millimeter sulcus depth is considered periodontal disease.
    A. One
    C. Three
    B. Two
    D. Six

16. Which charting color indicates work to be done? _____
    A. Black
    C. Blue
    B. Yellow
    D. Red

17. Which charting color indicates that work has been completed? _____
    A. Black
    C. Blue
    B. Yellow
    D. Red

18. What numbering system gives the primary teeth a letter or a "d" with a number? _____
    A. Fédération Dentaire Internationale
    B. Palmer
    C. Universal/National
    D. International Standards Organization

19. A(n) _____ restoration would be charted as outlined and filled in solidly with blue.
    A. gold   C. amalgam
    B. porcelain   D. composite

20. What restoration would be charted as outlined with swervy lines? _____
    A. gold crown   C. amalgam
    B. stainless steel D. composite

21. Composite restorations are charted by using which of the following charting schematics? _____
    A. Outlining
    B. Outlining and filling in
    C. Outlining with diagonal lines
    D. Crosshatch lines

22. A restoration charted as outlined with dots drawn would represent a(n) _____ restoration.
    A. amalgam   C. gold
    B. composite   D. porcelain

Cavity classifications aid in recording the type of dental caries. Match the cavity classification with the surface area(s).

Classification
23. _____ Class I
24. _____ Class II
25. _____ Class III
26. _____ Class IV
27. _____ Class V

Surface Area(s)
A. Two or more surfaces posterior
B. Interproximal surface of anterior
C. Cervical third facial or lingual surface
D. Caries in pit and fissures
E. Interproximal surface and incisal edge of anterior

There are several numbering systems. All patient records in one office are documented using one numbering system. Match the system with its corresponding coding.

System
28. _____ Universal/National
29. _____ Fédération Dentaire Internationale
30. _____ Palmer

Corresponding Coding
A. 1 for the upper right quadrant
B. 1–8 in each quadrant
C. 1–16, 17–32

Understanding the use of charting symbols is part of the accuracy of charting. Use the following charting conditions and match the corresponding charting symbol.

31. _____ Missing teeth
32. _____ Teeth impacted or unerupted
33. _____ Teeth that need root-canal therapy
34. _____ Tooth with full gold crown
35. _____ Tooth with porcelain crown

A.

B.

C.

D.

E.

CHAPTER 8

Microbiology

OBJECTIVES

The student should strive to meet the following objectives and demonstrate an understanding of the facts and principles presented in this chapter:

1. Identify Anton Van Leeuwenhoek, Louis Pasteur, and Robert Koch according to their contributions to microbiology.
2. Explain the groups of microorganisms and the staining procedures used to identify them.
3. Identify characteristics pertaining to the microorganism bacterium.
4. List characteristics pertaining to the microorganism protozoa.
5. Identify characteristics pertaining to the microorganism rickettsia.
6. Explain characteristics pertaining to the microorganisms yeasts and molds.
7. List characteristics pertaining to the microorganisms viruses.
8. Describe the diseases of major concern to the dental assistant and explain why they cause concern.
9. Identify how the body fights disease. Explain different immunities and routes of microorganism exposure.

SUMMARY

To safeguard against microorganism exposure in a dental office, one needs to understand how these pathogens pass from an infected person to a susceptible person. Therefore, within this chapter you will learn about pathogenic microorganisms along with the diseases they cause and how the body can defend against them.

KEY TERMS

acquired immunodeficiency
   syndrome (AIDS)
anaphylactic shock
antibodies
antigens

antitoxin
etiologic agent
human immunodeficiency virus
   (HIV)

pathogens
purulence
viral hepatitis

EXERCISES AND ACTIVITIES

1. The study of microorganisms is called _____
   A. pathogens. C. bacteria.
   B. microbiology. D. virus.

2. _____ was acknowledged for seeing microorganisms for the first time.
   A. Van Leeuwenhoek
   B. Pasteur
   C. Koch
   D. Rickettsia

3. _____ proved that bacteria caused disease.
   A. Van Leeuwenhoek
   B. Pasteur
   C. Koch
   D. Rickettsia

4. _____ determined the etiologic agent for tuberculosis.
   A. Van Leeuwenhoek
   B. Pasteur
   C. Koch
   D. Rickettsia

5. When a specific type of bacteria causes a specific disease this is called _____
   A. bacteria. C. spore.
   B. virus. D. etiologic.

6. A staining procedure to differentiate cells into two specific groups is called _____
   A. gram positive.
   B. Gram stain.
   C. gram negative.
   D. sporulating.

7. When Gram staining is demonstrated, if the cell wall keeps the color, the cells are classified as _____ _____ and appear dark purple under the microscope.
   A. gram negative
   B. gram positive

8. When Gram staining is demonstrated, if the cell wall loses color, the cells are classified as _____ _____ and appear colorless under the microscope.
   A. gram negative
   B. gram positive

9. _____ bacteria must have oxygen to grow and live.
   A. Anaerobic
   B. Facultative anaerobic
   C. Aerobic
   D. Sporulating

10. _____ bacteria will be destroyed in the presence of oxygen and live only without oxygen.
    A. Aerobic C. Facultative anaerobic
    B. Anaerobic D. Sporulating

11. _____ microorganisms under a microscope will appear rod shaped.
    A. Cocci C. Vibrios
    B. Spirilla D. Bacilli

12. _____ microorganisms under a microscope will appear round or bead shaped.
    A. Cocci C. Vibrios
    B. Spirilla D. Bacilli

13. Bacteria grown in colonies or clusters like grapes are called _____
    A. diplococci. C. streptococci.
    B. staphylococci. D. bacilli.

14. What mass of bacteria is identified by a chain shape or form? _____
    A. Diplococci D. Bacilli
    B. Staphylococci E. Maryland bridge
    C. Streptococci

15. Bacteria can cause various types of disease. Following is a list of symptoms. Which of these symptoms represent tuberculosis? _____
    1. Severe throat infection
    2. Tiredness
    3. Night sweats
    4. Whooping cough
    5. Persistent cough
    6. Stiffness of jaw

    A. 2, 3, 5
    B. 1, 2, 3
    C. 1, 3, 4
    D. 1, 4, 6

16. Name the group of bacteria that has been known to contribute to dental caries and endocarditis and lead to pneumonia or rheumatic fever. _____
    A. Staphylococcal
    B. Streptococcus mutans
    C. Bacilli
    D. Protozoa

17. _____ microorganisms are often referred to as amoebas and reproduce by binary fission.
    A. Staphylococcal
    B. Streptococcus mutans
    C. Bacilli
    D. Protozoa

18. Amebic dysentery is connected with which of the following? _____
    A. An infection
    B. Severe diarrhea is a symptom
    C. Can cause abscesses in liver
    D. Found in contaminated drinking water
    E. All of the above

19. The protozoa and bacteria microorganisms together cause a dental condition found in the inflamed tissue around the tooth, called _____
    A. dental decay.
    B. calculus/tartar.
    C. periodontal disease.
    D. candidiasis.

20. Two diseases caused by the Rickettsia microorganism are _____
    A. candidiasis and dysentery.
    B. malaria and periodontal disease.
    C. Rocky Mountain Spotted Fever and typhus.
    D. candidiasis and tinea.

21. Candidiasis is an infection caused by _____
    A. virus.
    B. fungus.
    C. influenza.
    D. herpes.

22. The fungal condition tinea corporis is commonly called _____
    A. athlete's foot.
    B. thrush.
    C. ringworm.
    D. measles.

23. _____ are the smallest microorganisms known to date and can be visualized only under an electron microscope.
    A. Bacteria
    B. Tinea
    C. Typhus
    D. Viruses

24. Which of the following are diseases caused by a virus? _____
    1. Measles
    2. Typhus
    3. Malaria
    4. Chicken pox
    5. Poliomyelitis
    6. Dysentery

    A. 1, 3, 6
    B. 1, 4, 5
    C. 1, 2, 3
    D. 2, 3, 6

25. What viral disease is usually associated with infections of the lips, mouth, and face? _____
    A. Herpetic whitlow
    B. Conjunctivitis
    C. Herpes simplex virus type 2
    D. Herpes simplex virus type 1

26. The _____ virus is extremely contagious and can spread by direct contact with the lesion or the fluid from the lesion.
    A. HIV
    B. hepatitis C
    C. herpes simplex
    D. hepatitis B

27. Which are high risk behaviors for acquiring hepatitis B? _____
    1. Injuries with sharp object contaminated with blood
    2. Usage of latex gloves
    3. Wearing a mask
    4. Multiple unprotected sexual partners
    5. Wearing eyewear
    6. Exposure to open wound with contaminated body fluid

    A. 1, 4, 5
    B. 2, 3, 5
    C. 1, 3, 6
    D. 1, 4, 6

28. Hepatitis _____ is transmitted by ingestion of contaminated food.
    A. E
    B. B
    C. A
    D. C

29. Hepatitis _____ is commonly called serum hepatitis.
    A. C   C. A
    B. B   D. C

30. Hepatitis _____ has a range of symptoms, including loss of appetite and jaundice.
    A. C   C. A
    B. B   D. C

31. The name of the current vaccine that shows effectiveness toward the hepatitis B virus is _____
    A. Heptavax-B.
    B. Recombivax HB.
    C. DPT.
    D. L-Lysen.

32. An individual who is a carrier of a disease but is not aware of it is called _____
    A. a Delta Agent.
    B. contaminate.
    C. asymptomatic.
    D. a case.

33. Name the retrovirus disease that attacks T-lymphocytes, part of the immune system, and multiplies. _____
    A. HBV   C. CDC
    B. HIV   D. MMR

34. Which of the following are full-blown AIDS conditions? _____
    1. Cancers
    2. Infections
    3. Diarrhea
    4. Constipation
    5. Lockjaw
    6. Rheumatic fever

    A. 3, 4, 5
    B. 1, 2, 3, 4, 5
    C. 1, 5, 6
    D. 3, 4, 6

35. A(n) _____ is a group of symptoms that characterize a disease.
    A. syndrome   C. spore
    B. etiologic agent   D. bacterium

36. The body responds to diseases in a number of ways. First, _____ must pass the body's first line of defense.
    A. antitoxins   C. antigens
    B. antibodies   D. pathogens

37. The _____ membrane is a wall that contains the infection and does not allow it to spread.
    A. periodontal   C. antigen
    B. pyogenic   D. toxin

38. As the body's final line of defense, _____ are formed to produce immunities against a foreign substance.
    A. antigens   C. antitoxins
    B. antibodies   D. pathogens

39. Pathogens that stimulate the production of antibodies are called _____
    A. antitoxins.   C. antigens.
    B. erythema.   D. allergens.

40. If immunity develops as a result of exposure to a pathogen, the immunity is called _____
    A. normal.   C. acquired.
    B. passive.   D. active.

41. An individual who has the ability to resist pathogens is called _____
    A. an allergen.   C. immune.
    B. hypersensitive.   D. erythemic.

42. If a person's antigen-antibody stimulates a massive secretion of histamine, the result would cause a severe reaction called _____
    A. active immunity.
    B. artificial immunity.
    C. passive immunity.
    D. anaphylactic shock.

43. If an antigen causes an allergic response, it is called _____
    A. immune   C. inoculated
    B. an allergen   D. hypersensitive

44. If a dental caregiver obtains a disease from a contaminated instrument, what route of exposure is this? _____
    A. Direct contact
    B. Indirect contact

Following are important people in microbiology. Match the name with the contribution.

Important People

45. _____ Anton Van Leeuwenhoek
46. _____ Louis Pasteur
47. _____ Robert Koch

Contribution

A. Proved that bacteria cause disease
B. Father of microbiology
C. Found that bacteria could be destroyed by heat

Following are groups of microorganisms. Match the organism with its disease or symptoms.

Microorganism

48. _____ Bacteria
49. _____ Protozoa
50. _____ Rickettsia
51. _____ Yeasts and molds
52. _____ Virus

Disease or Symptom

A. Amebic dysentery
B. MMR, poliomyelitis
C. Fungal infection
D. Typhus
E. TB, DPT

Following are diseases of major concern to the dental assistant. Match the disease with its infection.

Disease

53. _____ Herpes simplex virus type 1
54. _____ Herpes simplex virus type 2
55. _____ Hepatitis B
56. _____ HIV
57. _____ AIDS

Infection

A. Serum hepatitis
B. Class of retrovirus
C. Infections of lips, mouth, face
D. Infection that comes with HIV
E. Associated with genital area

Infection Control

The student should strive to meet the following objectives and demonstrate an understanding of the facts and principles presented in this chapter:

1. Identify the rationale, regulations, recommendations, and training that govern infection control in the dental office.
2. Describe how pathogens travel from person to person in the dental office.
3. List the three primary routes of microbial transmission and the associated dental procedures that affect the dental assistant.
4. Demonstrate the principles of infection control, including medical history, handwashing, personal protective equipment, barriers, chemical disinfectants, ultrasonic cleaners, sterilizers, and instrument storage.
5. List various disinfectants and their applications as used in dentistry.
6. Identify and demonstrate the usage of different types of sterilizers.
7. Demonstrate the usage of several types of sterilization monitors, such as biological and process indicators.
8. Identify and show the proper usage of pre-procedure mouth rinses, high volume evacuation, dental dams, and disposable items.
9. Identify and demonstrate the correct protocol for disinfecting, cleaning, and sterilizing prior to seating the patient, as well as at the end of the dental treatment, in the dental radiography area, and in the dental laboratory.

SUMMARY

Staff must be trained for a safe workplace. Compliance with all regulations must be accomplished to ensure that the process of infection control will be adequate. Training will occur at initial employment, when job tasks change, and annually thereafter.

KEY TERMS

American Dental Association
   (ADA)
antimicrobial
asepsis
aseptic technique
Bloodborne Pathogens Standard
Centers for Disease Control and
   Prevention (CDC)
contamination
direct contact
disinfect

Environmental Protection Agency
   (EPA)
Food and Drug Administration
   (FDA)
glutaraldehyde
indirect contact
infection control
inhalation
iodophor
Occupational Safety and Health
   Administration (OSHA)

other potentially infectious
   materials (OPIM)
pathogens
personal protective equipment
   (PPE)
polynitrile autoclavable
   gloves
standard precautions
sterilization
universal precautions

EXERCISES AND ACTIVITIES

1. _____ is the parent organization for dentistry in the United States.
   A. CDC
   B. OSHA
   C. United States Public Health Department
   D. ADA

2. Name the agency that is part of the Public Health Service, a division of the United States Department of Health and Human Services, and is the basis for many regulations. _____
   A. CDC
   B. OSHA
   C. ADA
   D. OPIM

3. _____ is a system that requires that PPE be worn to protect against contact with all body fluids, whether or not blood is visible.
   A. OSHA
   B. CDC
   C. OPIM
   D. Body substance isolation (BSI)

4. In compliance with infection control regulations, records must be maintained of staff for the duration of employment plus _____ years.
   A. seven
   B. ten
   C. thirty
   D. five

5. _____ precautions mean all patients are treated as if they are infectious.
   A. Universal
   B. OPIM
   C. FDA
   D. EPA

6. In 1992, OSHA established the Bloodborne Pathogens Standard, which mandates that facilities must do which of the following? _____
   1. Provide a sterile environment
   2. Protect workers from infectious hazards
   3. Provide automatic handwashing systems
   4. Provide antimicrobial soap
   5. Protect workers from chemical hazards
   6. Protect workers from physical hazards

   A. 1, 5, 6
   B. 2, 5, 6
   C. 2, 3, 4
   D. 1, 3, 4

7. An employee by job classification who would have any occupational exposure to blood would be a Category _____.
   A. 1
   B. 2
   C. 3
   D. 4

8. Items in the dental office, such as sterilizers and PPE, are regulated by the _____, which hold manufacturers responsible for problems that develop.
   A. ADA
   B. FDA
   C. EPA
   D. ADAA

9. Name the agency that regulates disposal of hazardous waste after it leaves the office. _____
   A. CDC
   B. OSHA
   C. FDA
   D. EPA

10. What cycle is perpetuated when pathogens are allowed to pass from dentist to patient or from patient to dentist? _____
    A. Material safety data
    B. Cross-contamination
    C. Pathogens Standard
    D. Standard exposure

11. If a dental assistant is hired, but the assistant has not had the hepatitis B immunization, who pays for the vaccine series? _____
    A. Dentist
    B. Assistant
    C. Accountant
    D. OSHA

12. It is important that the patient health history is updated at each appointment. Information should be updated both in writing and _____.
    A. by fax transmission
    B. over the phone
    C. verbally
    D. by e-mail

13. Patients could be infected with HBV and HIV and have no symptoms. This condition is called _____.
    A. cross-contamination
    B. antimicrobial
    C. asymptomatic
    D. transient

14. One of the primary concerns of handwashing is to remove the _____ microorganisms because they constitute the group that includes hepatitis.
    A. transient
    B. causative
    C. bloodborne
    D. saliva

15. During the handwashing procedure, proper chemical antisepsis is accomplished with _____
    A. chlorhexidine digluconate.
    B. triclosan.
    C. para-chlorometaxylenol.
    D. All of the above

16. The minimal handwash before and after patient care is _____ seconds.
    A. sixty   C. fifteen
    B. thirty   D. ninety

17. Barriers to prevent potential pathogens, encountered during patient care, from gaining access to dental personnel include which of the following? _____
    1. Material safety data sheets (MSDS)
    2. EPA
    3. Regulations
    4. Gloves
    5. Mask
    6. Eyewear

    A. 1, 2, 3
    B. 4, 5, 6
    C. 1, 4, 5
    D. 2, 3, 5

18. _____ developed a standard for the design and characteristics of occupational glasses.
    A. CDC   C. EPA
    B. OSHA   D. ANSI

19. _____ regulates the gloves specific for the healthcare industry.
    A. FDA   C. OSHA
    B. EPA   D. CDC

20. _____ gloves are used for patient treatment any time the dental assistant anticipates contact with saliva or blood.
    A. Polynitrile   C. Utility
    B. Nitrile   D. Vinyl

21. _____ are worn by dental assistants any time there is the possibility of aerosol mist.
    A. Overgloves   C. Rubber dams
    B. Masks   D. Lead aprons

22. The dental _____ also protects the patient and assistant from the transmission of communicable diseases.
    A. handpiece   C. mask
    B. scaler   D. ultrasonic

23. Special protective clothing worn only in the dental office is regulated by OSHA and includes _____
    A. uniforms.
    B. lab coats.
    C. gowns.
    D. Clinic jackets.
    E. All of the above

24. When the gown or uniform is on, the glove fits _____ it.
    A. over   B. under

25. Special protective clothing is regulated by OSHA. Which of the following are OSHA regulations regarding special protective clothing? _____
    1. Worn only in the dental offices
    2. Can be changed weekly
    3. Must be laundered in office or a laundry service
    4. Must close tightly at neck and around cuff
    5. Must be knee length when sitting during high-risk procedure
    6. Must bear ornamental designs
    7. Must be removed if going out to lunch or into lunch room
    8. Must be removed at end of day prior to going home
    9. Gown can be short-sleeved for summer
    10. Cuffs of gown do not need to overlap with cuffs of gloves

    A. 2, 5, 6, 8, 9, 10
    B. 1, 3, 6, 7, 9, 10
    C. 1, 3, 4, 5, 7, 8
    D. 2, 3, 7, 8, 9, 10

26. Concerning the requirement of asepsis, some surfaces do not lend themselves to the use of barriers. Those surfaces will need to be _____
    A. suctioned.   C. autoclaved.
    B. sterilized.   D. disinfected.

27. According to the EPA ratings, the disinfection level that will kill most bacterial spores is _____
    A. high.   C. low.
    B. intermediate. D. holding.

28. Which of the following is considered the high-level disinfectant? _____
    A. Alcohol   C. Iodopher
    B. Glutaraldehyde D. Sodium hypochlorite

29. Which of the following is considered the intermediate-level disinfectant? _____
    A. Alcohol   C. Glutaraldehyde
    B. Chlorine dioxide D. Iodopher

30. The device that uses sound waves that travel through glass and metal using a special solution to clean debris from dental instruments is the _____
    A. sterilizer.   C. ultrasonic cleaner.
    B. autoclave.   D. holding bath.

31. All forms of microorganisms are destroyed in the process of _____.
    - A. disinfection
    - C. sterilization
    - B. asepsis
    - D. sanitization

32. If immersion sterilization is used, items are placed in the disinfecting solution for _____ hour(s) to ensure that all microorganisms are destroyed.
    - A. one
    - C. ten
    - B. five
    - D. three

33. Name the sterilizer that operates at approximately 450°F. _____
    - A. Dry heat
    - B. Chemical vapor
    - C. Ethylene oxide
    - D. Glass bead

34. Most dental offices sterilize their dental handpiece exclusively in the _____ _____ sterilizer.
    - A. chemical vapor
    - B. dry heat
    - C. steam autoclave
    - D. glass bead

35. _____ monitors offer the most accurate way to assess that sterilization has occurred.
    - A. Cavitation
    - C. Cleaning
    - B. Biological
    - D. Sanitizing

36. _____ indicators are printed on packaging materials for sterilization and contain dyes that change color upon quick exposure to sterilizing cycles.
    - A. Biological
    - C. Sanitizing
    - B. Process
    - D. Disinfecting

37. _____ indicators are placed inside sterilization packing and indicate whether the correct conditions were present for sterilization to take place.
    - A. Biological
    - C. Process
    - B. Dosage
    - D. Disinfecting

38. What pre-procedure reduces the total number of microorganisms in the oral cavity? _____
    - A. Antiseptic mouth rinse
    - B. Rubber dam
    - C. Evacuation system
    - D. Disinfectant

39. If an acrylic appliance needs to be sent from the dental office to an outside lab, the appliance will need to be placed into _____
    - A. diluted sodium hypochlorite.
    - B. dry heat.
    - C. chemical vapor.
    - D. steam.

To provide complete infection control in a dental office, a number of steps must be followed. Match the following standards with the protection they provide both the patient and assistant.

Standard

40. _____ Immunization
41. _____ Handwashing
42. _____ Protective eyewear
43. _____ Gloves
44. _____ Mask

Protection Benefit

- A. Meets ANSI requirements
- B. Protects the mucous membrane from aerosol
- C. Hepatitis B vaccine
- D. Removes transient microorganisms
- E. Five primary types and are regulated by FDA

Numerous gloves are available that meet FDA regulations. Following are four of the primary types of gloves. Match the glove with its designed use for the dental team member.

Glove Type

45. _____ Latex
46. _____ Overglove
47. _____ Utility
48. _____ Polynitrile

Glove Use

- A. Known as food handlers' glove
- B. Can be washed and reused
- C. Can be sterilized in autoclave after each use
- D. Referred to as examination glove

To ensure that all items used in intraoral procedures are sterile, there are several sterilization choices available. Match the sterilization method with its use.

Sterilization Method

49. _____ Liquid chemical disinfectant
50. _____ Ethylene oxide
51. _____ Dry heat
52. _____ Chemical vapor
53. _____ Steam autoclave

Use

- A. Uses heat 340°F
- B. Uses 250°F
- C. Requires ten hours in solution
- D. Uses 120°F
- E. Must be 270°F

SKILL COMPETENCY ASSESSMENT

9-1 Handwashing

Student's Name _____ Date _____

Instructor's Name _____

SKILL   At the beginning of each day, two consecutive thirty-second handwashings should be performed. This should consist of a vigorous rubbing together of well-lathered soapy hands (ensuring friction on all surfaces), concluding with a thorough rinsing under a stream of water and proper drying. Handwashing is both a mechanical cleaning and chemical antisepsis.

PERFORMANCE OBJECTIVE   The student will remove jewelry, adjust the water flow and wet hands thoroughly, apply antimicrobial soap, and bring to a lather while rubbing all areas of the hands, getting between fingers and cleaning beneath finger nails. Rinse and dry thoroughly.

	Self Evaluation	Student Evaluation	Possible Points	Instructor Evaluation	Comments
Equipment and Supplies					
1. Liquid antimicrobial handwashing agent			1		
2. Soft, sterile brush or sponge (optional)			1		
3. Sink with hot and cold running water			1		
4. Paper towels			1		
Competency Steps					
1. Remove jewelry (rings and watch).			2		
2. Adjust water flow and wet hands thoroughly.			2		
3. Apply antimicrobial handwashing agents with water; bring to a lather.			2		
4. Scrub hands together or with a sterile brush or sponge, making sure to get between each finger, the surface of the palms and wrists, and under the finger nails.			3		
5. Rinse and repeat Steps 3 and 4.			2		
6. Final rinse with cool to lukewarm water for ten seonds to close the pores.			1		
7. Dry with paper towels, the hands first and then the wrist area.			1		
8. Use paper towels to turn off the hand-controlled faucets.			2		

TOTAL POINTS POSSIBLE   19

TOTAL POINTS POSSIBLE—2nd Attempt   17

TOTAL POINTS EARNED   _____

Points assigned reflect importance of step to meeting objective: Important = 1; Essential = 2; Critical = 3. Students will lose 2 points for repeated attempts. Failure results if any of the critical steps are omitted or performed incorrectly. If using a 100-point scale, determine score by dividing points earned by total points possible and multiplying the results by 100.

SCORE: _____

SKILL COMPETENCY ASSESSMENT

|9-2 Preparing the Dental Treatment Room

Student's Name _____ Date _____

Instructor's Name _____

SKILL Routine steps should be followed for all treatment areas to maintain absolute clinical asepsis.

PERFORMANCE OBJECTIVE The student will follow a routine procedure that meets the regulations and the protocol set forth by the dentist and regulatory agencies. The dental assistant prepares the operatory and equipment.

	Self Evaluation	Student Evaluation	Possible Points	Instructor Evaluation	Comments
Equipment and Supplies					
1. Patient's medical and dental history (including dental radiographs)			2		
2. Barriers for dental chair, hoses, counter, light switches, and controls			3		
3. PPE for dental assistant (protective eyewear, mask, gloves, and overgloves)			3		
4. Patient napkin, napkin chain, and protective eyewear			3		
5. Sterile procedure tray			3		
Competency Steps					
1. Wash hands.			3		
2. Review the patient's medical and dental history, place radiographs on viewbox, and identify procedure to be completed at this visit. Patient's medical and dental history can be placed in a plastic envelope or under a surface barrier.			3		
3. Place new barriers on all possible surfaces that can be contaminated (for example, dental chair, hoses, counter, light switches, and controls).			3		
4. Bring the instrument tray with packaged sterile instruments into the operatory with patient's napkin and protective eyewear.			3		
5. Prepare dental assistant PPE (protective eyewear, mask, gloves, and overgloves).			3		

TOTAL POINTS POSSIBLE 29

TOTAL POINTS POSSIBLE—2nd Attempt 27

TOTAL POINTS EARNED _____

Points assigned reflect importance of step to meeting objective: Important = 1; Essential = 2; Critical = 3. Students will lose 2 points for repeated attempts. Failure results if any of the critical steps are omitted or performed incorrectly. If using a 100-point scale, determine score by dividing points earned by total points possible and multiplying the results by 100.

SCORE: _____

SKILL COMPETENCY ASSESSMENT

9-3 Completion of Dental Treatment

Student's Name _____ Date _____

Instructor's Name _____

SKILL Routine steps should be followed for all treatment areas upon completion of dental treatment. Maintain absolute clinical asepsis and prevent cross-contamination.

PERFORMANCE OBJECTIVE The student will follow a routine procedure that meets the regulations and the protocol set forth by the dentist and regulatory agencies. The dental assistant completes the procedure and dismisses the patient.

	Self Evaluation	Student Evaluation	Possible Points	Instructor Evaluation	Comments
Equipment and Supplies					
1. Patient's medical and dental history (including dental radiographs)			3		
2. Barriers for dental chair, hoses, counter, light switches, and controls			3		
3. Dental handpiece			1		
4. Air-water syringe tip (disposable)			1		
5. Patient napkin			1		
6. Contaminated instruments on tray, including HVE tip			3		
Competency Steps					
1. Remove handpieces, HVE tip, and air-water tip and place on treatment tray.			3		
2. Place on overgloves to document on chart or on the computer and assemble radiographs and chart, preventing cross-contamination.			3		
3. Remove patient napkin and place over the treatment tray prior to dismissing the patient.			1		
With gloves in place, complete the following:					
4. Place the handpiece, HVE, and air-water syringe back on unit and run for twenty to thirty seconds to clean the lines or flush the system. Remove handpiece and air-water syringe and place back on the treatment tray.			3		
5. Place sharps into puncture-resistant sharps disposal containers.			3		
6. Remove chair cover from the patient dental chair, inverting it so that any splatter or debris remains inside the bag.			1		
7. Removal all the barriers and place them in inverted bag. Any disposables can be placed in the bag as well.			2		

9-3 continued

	Self Evaluation	Student Evaluation	Possible Points	Instructor Evaluation	Comments
8. Carry treatment tray with all items from the treatment area to sterilizing area. Nothing left in operatory at this time that is to be sterilized.			2		
9. Remove the treatment gloves and place them in the inverted bag. Dispose of the bag.			1		
10. Wash hands.			1		

TOTAL POINTS POSSIBLE   32

TOTAL POINTS POSSIBLE—2nd Attempt   30

TOTAL POINTS EARNED   _____

Points assigned reflect importance of step to meeting objective: Important = 1; Essential = 2; Critical = 3. Students will lose 2 points for repeated attempts. Failure results if any of the critical steps are omitted or performed incorrectly. If using a 100-point scale, determine score by dividing points earned by total points possible and multiplying the results by 100.

SCORE: _____

SKILL COMPETENCY ASSESSMENT

9-4 Final Treatment Room Disinfecting and Cleaning

Student's Name _____ Date _____

Instructor's Name _____

SKILL The process of cleaning (physical removal of organic matter such as blood, tissue, and debris) decreases the number of microorganisms in the area and removes substances that may hinder the process of disinfection. As long as all surfaces are disinfected, the requirements of asepsis are met.

PERFORMANCE OBJECTIVE The student will follow a routine procedure that meets the regulations and the protocol set forth by the dentist and regulatory agencies. The dental assistant completes the procedure for disinfecting and cleaning after the treatment has been completed and the patient has been dismissed.

	Self Evaluation	Student Evaluation	Possible Points	Instructor Evaluation	Comments
Equipment and Supplies					
1. Utility gloves			2		
2. Necessary disinfecting solutions (intermediate level)			2		
3. Wiping cloths			1		
4. 4 x 4 gauze			1		
Competency Steps					
1. Wash hands, place on utility gloves. • Obtain necessary solutions/wiping cloths • 4 x 4 gauze (items could be in a small utility carry tote)			2		
2. All surfaces need to be sprayed and cleaned first, then wiped to remove debris.			2		
3. The initial spray wipe can be done by using saturated "wiping devices" (prepare by spraying 4 x 4 gauze with disinfectant) and wiping each surface carefully/thoroughly.			2		
4. Spray on the disinfectant and leave for the correct time to accomplish disinfection (normally ten minutes).			2		
5. Rewipe all surfaces.			3		
6. Review that all surfaces that could have been contaminated are disinfected (amalgam cradle, chair adjustments, curing light, radiographic viewbox switch).			2		

TOTAL POINTS POSSIBLE   19

TOTAL POINTS POSSIBLE—2nd Attempt   17

TOTAL POINTS EARNED   _____

Points assigned reflect importance of step to meeting objective: Important = 1; Essential = 2; Critical = 3. Students will lose 2 points for repeated attempts. Failure results if any of the critical steps are omitted or performed incorrectly. If using a 100-point scale, determine score by dividing points earned by total points possible and multiplying the results by 100.

SCORE: _____

SKILL COMPETENCY ASSESSMENT

|9-5 Treatment of Contaminated Tray in the Sterilization Center

Student's Name _____ Date _____

Instructor's Name _____

SKILL Once the treatment tray has been removed from the operatory and into the sterilization center, the dental assistant is ready to process the instruments. At this time, all the debris, blood, saliva, and tissue are removed from the instruments to ensure that sterilization can be completed on all surfaces.

PERFORMANCE OBJECTIVE The student will follow a routine procedure that meets the regulations and the protocol set forth by the dentist and regulatory agencies. The dental assistant completes the procedure in the sterilization center.

	Self Evaluation	Student Evaluation	Possible Points	Instructor Evaluation	Comments
Equipment and Supplies					
1. Utility gloves			2		
2. Necessary disinfecting solutions			2		
3. Wiping cloths			1		
4. 4 x 4 gauze			1		
5. Contaminated procedure tray			1		
Competency Steps					
1. Place treatment tray in contaminated area of sterilization center. Return later for processing.			2		
2. Place instruments into holding solution as soon as possible to prevent debris from drying.			2		
3. Wear utility gloves during the entire procedure of caring for contaminated instrument tray.			3		
4. Place sharps into sharps container if not already accomplished in the dental operatory.			2		
5. All disposable items are discarded. Biohazard waste must be placed in an appropriately labeled waste container.			3		
6. Instruments from the holding solution are rinsed and placed into the ultrasonic cleaner. Small strainers will hold small items (burs, dental dam clamps). After the timed cleaning is completed (usually three to ten minutes), rinse items thoroughly.			3		
7. After rinsing the instruments, towel dry, bag, date, and place into appropriate sterilizer. If cassette is used versus bagging, instruments can be dipped into alcohol bath and left to air dry before placing in sealed bag and in sterilizer.			3		
8. Dental high-speed handpiece is rinsed off with isopropyl alcohol, lubricated, bagged in an instrument pouch, and placed in appropriate sterilizer (follow manufacturer's directions).			3		

9-5 continued

	Self Evaluation	Student Evaluation	Possible Points	Instructor Evaluation	Comments
9. The instrument tray and other items left on tray need to be spray wiped, sprayed again, left for ten minutes (follow manufacturer's directions), and wiped again before assembling them for another tray setup.			2		
10. Clean up area used in the sterilization center, wash and dry utility gloves, remove them, and wash and dry hands.			1		
11. When sterilizer indicates that the instruments are sterile, the pressure is released, and the door or tray is opened. The instruments can be removed from the sterilizer with forceps.			3		

TOTAL POINTS POSSIBLE   34

TOTAL POINTS POSSIBLE—2nd Attempt   32

TOTAL POINTS EARNED   _____

Points assigned reflect importance of step to meeting objective: Important = 1; Essential = 2; Critical = 3. Students will lose 2 points for repeated attempts. Failure results if any of the critical steps are omitted or performed incorrectly. If using a 100-point scale, determine score by dividing points earned by total points possible and multiplying the results by 100.

SCORE: _____

Management of Hazardous Materials

OBJECTIVES

The student should strive to meet the following objectives and demonstrate an understanding of the facts and principles presented in this chapter:

1. Identify the scope of the OSHA Bloodborne/Hazardous Materials Standard.
2. Identify physical equipment and mechanical devices provided to safeguard employees.
3. Demonstrate disposal of sharps.
4. Describe MSDS manuals.
5. Demonstrate the use of the colors and numbers used for hazardous chemical identification.
6. Describe employee training required to meet the OSHA standard for hazardous chemicals.

SUMMARY

The Occupational Safety and Health Administration regulations, including the hazard communication standard, are intended to require the employer to provide a safe work environment for all employees. The dental assistant must understand the complete standard and how compliance is accomplished. Staff must be trained for a safe workplace. Compliance with all standards must be accomplished to ensure a safe workplace.

KEY TERMS

material safety data sheets (MSDS)
National Fire Protection Association's color and number method

Occupational Safety and Health Administration (OSHA)
other potentially infectious material (OPIM)
parenteral

pericardial
peritoneal
pleural
synovial

EXERCISES AND ACTIVITIES

1. Employees in the dental office need to know and comply with the OSHA safety standards. Which of the following is not an OSHA safety standard? _____
   A. Employee training
   B. Labeling/MSDS
   C. Housekeeping/laundry
   D. ADA

2. The physical equipment and mechanical devices that employers provide to safeguard and protect employees are known as _____
   A. material safety data sheets.
   B. engineering/work practice controls.
   C. housekeeping/laundry.
   D. labeling.

3. Which of the following items are considered engineering/work practice controls? _____
   1. Splash guards on model trimmers
   2. Puncture-resistant sharps containers
   3. Etiologic agent
   4. Ventilation hoods for hazardous fumes
   5. Eye-wash station
   6. Gram stain
   7. Amebic dysentery
   8. Tinea

   A. 1, 2, 4, 5
   B. 3, 6, 7, 8
   C. 3, 4, 6, 7
   D. 1, 2, 3, 5

4. Which of the following is not included in the definition of human fluids as blood? _____
   A. Blood and anything that is visually contaminated with blood
   B. Saliva in dental oral procedures
   C. Synovial fluid
   D. Distilled water

5. _____ is a means of piercing mucous membranes or the skin barrier.
   A. OPIM   C. Synovial
   B. Parenteral   D. Biohazardous

6. Which of the following would not go into the sharps? _____
   A. Orthodontic wire
   B. Contaminated needles
   C. Surgical knives or blades
   D. Rubber dam

7. The sharps container must meet very strict standards. Which of the following descriptors is not part of the sharps standard? _____
   A. Labeled
   B. Leakproof
   C. Wide-mouth opening
   D. Puncture resistant

8. If an occupational exposure occurs, which of the following is(are) required for any employee? _____
   A. The employee must report the incident immediately.
   B. Employer must immediately provide medical evaluation and follow-up.
   C. Medical evaluation and follow-up are made available to employee at no cost.
   D. The dentist evaluates the circumstances surrounding the incident and finds ways to prevent it from happening again.
   E. All of the above

9. Documentation of an exposure incident must include testing for _____
   A. tetanus.   C. HBV.
   B. MMR.   D. TB.

10. If employees choose to decline testing after an exposure incident, they can delay testing up to _____ days.
    A. ninety   C. thirty
    B. sixty   D. twenty-eight

11. A post-exposure prophylaxis is provided according to the current recommendations of _____
    A. OSHA.
    B. United States Public Health Service.
    C. CDC.
    D. ADA.

12. In accordance with OSHA's standard on Access to Employee Exposure and Medical Records, the employer must maintain employee records for _____ year(s).
    A. fifteen   C. one
    B. twenty-four   D. thirty

13. Gloves that are contaminated with blood are required to go into _____
    A. regular waste.
    B. a biohazard container.
    C. the laundry.
    D. leak-proof sharps.

14. The type of gloves worn while cleaning or disinfecting contaminated surfaces is _____
    A. vinyl.   C. surgical.
    B. latex.   D. utility.

15. _____ regulations ensure a safe work environment regarding the risks of using hazardous chemicals.
    A. ADA   C. OSHA
    B. EPA   D. Bloodborne

16. Within _____ days of employment, employee training must occur regarding the identification of hazardous chemicals and personal protective equipment that will be utilized.
    A. ninety   C. thirty
    B. fifteen   D. sixty

17. The _____ color and number method is used to signify a warning to employees using chemicals.
    A. Centers for Disease Control
    B. National Fire Protection Association
    C. Occupational Safety and Health Administration
    D. American Dental Association

18. The color _____ identifies the health hazard.
    A. red   C. white
    B. yellow   D. blue

OSHA and the CDC define these human fluids as blood. Match the fluid with its excretion.

Fluid
19. _____ Synovial
20. _____ Saliva
21. _____ Pleural
22. _____ Peritoneal
23. _____ Pericardial

Excretion
A. Abdominal fluid
B. Heart fluid
C. Joint and tendon fluid
D. Intraoral dental
E. Lung fluid

The National Fire Protection Association's color method is used to signify a warning to employees using chemicals. Match the color with its hazard.

Color
24. _____ Blue
25. _____ Red
26. _____ Yellow
27. _____ White

Hazard
A. Reactivity or stability
B. Health
C. PPE needed
D. Fire

Preparation for Patient Care

The student should strive to meet the following objectives and demonstrate an understanding of the facts and principles presented in this chapter:

1. Assist the patient in completing the patient history.
2. Review the medical and dental history. Alert the dentist to any areas of concerns.
3. Perform or assist the dentist in an oral evaluation, including lips, tongue, glands, and oral cavity.
4. Perform vital signs on the patient, including temperature, pulse, respiration, and blood pressure.
5. Read the vital signs. Alert the dentist if they are abnormal.

SUMMARY

The health condition of a dental patient must be private, confidential, and updated at each visit. To treat a patient effectively, the patient's chart should include personal history, medical information, dental history, clinical observation, clinical evaluation, and vital signs.

KEY TERMS

antipyretic	diastolic blood pressure	sphygmomanometer
asymmetric	exhalation	stethoscope
baseline vital signs	Fahrenheit	symmetric
brachial artery	fever	systolic blood pressure
bradycardia	hypothermic	tachycardia
bradypnea	inhalation	tachypnea
Celsius	palpates	vermilion border
commissures	smile line	vital signs

EXERCISES AND ACTIVITIES

1. A patient is requested to fill out a personal history questionnaire. Which of the following is not a part of this history? _____
   A. Full name   C. Address
   B. Vital signs   D. Phone number

2. Which of the following health history questions is critical in that it could affect treatment? _____
   A. Surgeries   C. Injuries
   B. Systemic diseases D. Allergies

3. Which of the following allergies would concern the dentist as it related to patient treatment? _____
   A. Anesthetics   C. Dental phobia
   B. Amalgams   D. Surgeries

4. If a patient indicates an epileptic condition, this information would be found in what section of the patient's chart? _____
   A. Personal
   B. Medical history
   C. Vital response
   D. Clinical observation

5. The dentist has a _____ responsibility to gain information about a patient's medical history prior to dental treatment.
   A. clinical   C. health
   B. legal   D. personal

6. The dental assistant can observe patients as they are escorted to the treatment room and can note which of the following? _____
   A. Walk or gait
   B. Speech
   C. Facial symmetry
   D. Eyes
   E. All of the above

7. The vermilion border is defined as _____
   A. smile line.
   B. commissures.
   C. line around the lips.
   D. cracking or dryness.

8. The area of the neck from the ear to the collar bone that is examined during the external clinical examination is called the _____
   A. TMJ.
   B. floor of the mouth.
   C. lips.
   D. lymph nodes.

9. During the clinical exam, what area does the dental assistant palpate as the patient opens and closes the mouth? _____
   A. TMJ
   B. Floor of the mouth
   C. Lips
   D. Lymph nodes

10. Which of the following is not assessed during an internal oral examination? _____
    A. Lesions in the mouth
    B. Abscessed teeth
    C. Color changes in oral mucosa
    D. Noise from clicking or catching in jaw
    E. Ventral sides of tongue

11. The basic signs of life are called the _____
    A. pulse.
    B. respiration rate.
    C. vital signs.
    D. body temperature.

12. An adult average baseline body temperature is _____
    A. 99.5°F.   C. 96.0°F.
    B. 98.6°F.   D. 37.5°C.

13. Body temperature can vary from patient to patient and at different times of the day. Which of the following can cause an increase in temperature? _____
    A. Exercise
    B. Eating
    C. Emotional excitement
    D. Blushing or turning red
    E. All of the above

14. When a manual thermometer is used, it will be placed _____
    A. between buccal mucosa.
    B. only between the lips.
    C. under the tongue.
    D. None of the above

15. If a digital thermometer is used to obtain a patient's temperature, how should the probe cover be disposed of? _____
    A. Regular waste
    B. Biohazard waste

16. Which is not a recorded pulse site? _____
    A. Radial   C. Carotid
    B. TMJ   D. Temporial

17. Respiration is one breath taken in, called _____,
    and one breath let out.
    A. tachypnea   C. exhalation
    B. bradypnea   D. inhalation

18. Normal pulse rate for adults is _____
    A. 90 to 120 beats per minute.
    B. 12 to 18 beats per minute.
    C. 60 to 90 beats per minute.
    D. 20 to 40 beats per minute.

19. Normal respiration rate for children is _____
    A. 90 to 120 respirations per minute.
    B. 12 to 18 respirations per minute.
    C. 60 to 90 respirations per minute.
    D. 20 to 40 respirations per minute.

20. Blood pressure is an important indicator of
    a patient's _____
    A. dental condition.
    B. cardiovascular condition.
    C. body temperature.
    D. respiration rate.

21. The brachial artery is located _____
    A. inside the wrist.
    B. under the chin.
    C. in the neck area.
    D. inside the elbow.

22. What piece of blood pressure equipment is placed
    above the bend of the elbow and secured? _____
    A. Stethoscope
    B. Sphygmomanometer

23. The blood pressure cuff is placed _____ inch(es)
    above the bend of the elbow and secured.
    A. two   C. three
    B. one   D. four

24. The stethoscope earpieces must be placed in the
    ears in a _____ position.
    A. forward
    B. distal

25. Normal blood pressure range for an adult is _____
    A. 100 to 140 mm Hg/60 to 90 mm Hg.
    B. 60 to 100 mm Hg/33 to 66 mm Hg.
    C. 68 to 118 mm Hg/46 to 76 mm Hg.
    D. None of the above

Body temperature is an essential component of every patient.
Match the term with its use.

Term

26. _____ Fever
27. _____ Hypothermic
28. _____ Antipyretic
29. _____ Fahrenheit

Use

A. Used to reduce fever
B. Above the normal temperature range
C. Measure of temperature
D. Below the normal temperature range

The pulse is another component of the patient's vital signs.
Match the term with the best definition.

Term

30. _____ Pulse
31. _____ Radial site
32. _____ Carotid site
33. _____ Temporal site

Definition

A. Front of ear/level of eyebrow
B. Large artery in neck
C. Thumb side of wrist
D. Intermittent beating sensation

Respiration is another vital sign of record. Match the term with the best definition.

Term

34. _____ Inhalation
35. _____ Exhalation
36. _____ Tachypnea
37. _____ Bradypnea

Definition

A. Abnormally slow resting rate
B. One breath taken in
C. One breath let out
D. Abnormally rapid resting rate

Blood pressure is an important indicator of the health of a patient's cardiovascular system. Match the term with the definition.

Term

38. _____ Sphygmomanometer
39. _____ Brachial artery
40. _____ Stethoscope
41. _____ Systolic pressure
42. _____ Diastolic pressure

Definition

A. First sound as heart contracts blood through arteries
B. Inflatable bladder to control blood flow to artery
C. Pulsation sound disappears as arteries relax
D. Instrument used to hear and amplify sounds of heart
E. First palpated inside of elbow

SKILL COMPETENCY ASSESSMENT

11-1 Taking a Radial Pulse and Measuring the Respiration Rate
(corresponds to textbook Procedure 11-2)

Student's Name _____ Date _____

Instructor's Name _____

SKILL To identify body pulse and respiration compared to the normal rates for every patient health evaluation. Rates will vary depending on the patient's age, sex, and physical and mental condition.

PERFORMANCE OBJECTIVE The student will follow a routine procedure that meets the guidelines and protocol to obtain the patient's vital signs. The dental assistant completes the procedure in the dental operatory.

	Self Evaluation	Student Evaluation	Possible Points	Instructor Evaluation	Comments
Equipment and Supplies					
1. Watch with a second hand			3		
Competency Steps					
1. Wash hands.			2		
2. Position patient in a comfortable, upright position (same as for temperature).			2		
3. Explain procedure.			3		
4. Have patient position the wrist resting on arm of dental chair or counter.			2		
5. Locate the radial pulse by placing the pads of the first three fingers over the patient's wrist.			3		
6. Gently compress the radial artery so that the pulse can be felt.			2		
7. Using the watch with the second hand, count the number of pulsations for one full minute.			2		
8. Record the number of pulsations.			2		
9. Note any irregular rhythm patterns.			2		
10. While keeping finger pads placed on the radial pulse, count the rise and fall of the chest for one minute.			2		
11. Record the number of respirations. Note any irregularities in the breathing.			2		
12. Wash hands.			1		
13. Document the procedure and the pulse and respiration rate on the patient's chart.			2		

TOTAL POINTS POSSIBLE   30

TOTAL POINTS POSSIBLE—2nd Attempt   28

TOTAL POINTS EARNED   _____

Points assigned reflect importance of step to meeting objective: Important = 1; Essential = 2; Critical = 3. Students will lose 2 points for repeated attempts. Failure results if any of the critical steps are omitted or performed incorrectly. If using a 100-point scale, determine score by dividing points earned by total points possible and multiplying the results by 100.

SCORE: _____

SKILL COMPETENCY ASSESSMENT

11-2 Measuring Blood Pressure *(corresponds to textbook Procedure 11-3)*

Student's Name _____ Date _____

Instructor's Name _____

SKILL Identifying the patient's blood pressure compared to the normal blood pressure is an important indicator of a patient's health. Blood pressures will vary in ranges much like other vital signs. Children normally have lower pressure; as adults age, the blood pressure goes up.

PERFORMANCE OBJECTIVE The student will follow a routine procedure that meets the guidelines and protocol to obtain the patient's blood pressure. The dental assistant completes the procedure in the dental operatory.

	Self Evaluation	Student Evaluation	Possible Points	Instructor Evaluation	Comments
Equipment and Supplies					
1. Stethoscope			2		
2. Sphygmomanometer			2		
3. Disinfectant and gauze			1		
Competency Steps					
1. Wash hands.			2		
2. Assemble the stethoscope and the sphygmomanometer and disinfect the earpieces of the stethoscope.			3		
3. Position the patient in a comfortable position, upright in the dental chair (same as for temperature).			1		
4. Explain procedure.			2		
5. Have patient position arm resting at heart level on the counter or the arm of dental chair.			2		
6. Have the patient remove any outer clothing that is restrictive to upper arm. Bare the upper arm and palpate the brachial artery.			2		
7. Center the bladder of the cuff securely, about two inches above the bend of the elbow.			2		
8. Position the earpieces of stethoscope in a forward manner into the ears.			2		
9. Place diaphragm of stethoscope over brachial artery, holding in place with thumb. Place other fingers under the elbow to hyperextend the artery (access is easier and enables better reading).			3		
10. Inflate the cuff using bulb and the control valve of sphygmomanometer. If cuff is not inflating, recheck control valve on sphygmomanometer to ensure it is closed. Air should not escape. Inflation level should be 160 for a normal adult.			3		

11-2 continued *(corresponds to textbook Procedure 11-3)*

	Self Evaluation	Student Evaluation	Possible Points	Instructor Evaluation	Comments
11. Deflate cuff at a rate of two to four millimeters of mercury per second by rotating control valve slightly.			3		
12. Listen for first sound and note its measurement on the scale.			1		
13. Continue to deflate the cuff and listen to the pulsing sounds. Note when all sounds disappear. Continue deflating for another ten millimeters to ensure the last sound has been heard.			2		
14. The cuff can then be deflated rapidly and removed from patient's arm.			3		
15. Disinfect the earpieces of stethoscope.			1		
16. Wash hands and record the procedure and the measurement on the patient's chart. (Blood pressure is recorded in even numbers in a fraction format with the systolic measurement on top.)			3		

TOTAL POINTS POSSIBLE   40

TOTAL POINTS POSSIBLE—2nd Attempt   38

TOTAL POINTS EARNED   _____

Points assigned reflect importance of step to meeting objective: Important = 1; Essential = 2; Critical = 3. Students will lose 2 points for repeated attempts. Failure results if any of the critical steps are omitted or performed incorrectly. If using a 100-point scale, determine score by dividing points earned by total points possible and multiplying the results by 100.

SCORE: _____

Pharmacology

OBJECTIVES

The student should strive to meet the following objectives and demonstrate an understanding of the facts and principles presented in this chapter:

1. Identify the terms related to drugs, pharmacology, and medicines.
2. Identify the difference between drug brand names and generic names.
3. Identify the parts of a written prescription.
4. Identify the texts pertinent to pharmacology.
5. Give the English meanings of the Latin abbreviations used for prescriptions.
6. Specify the drug laws and who enforces them.
7. Identify the schedules for the Comprehensive Drug Abuse Prevention and Control Act of 1970.
8. Identify the routes in which drugs can be administered.
9. Summarize the uses and effects of tobacco, caffeine, alcohol, marijuana, and cocaine.
10. Summarize information about heroin, morphine, and codeine.
11. Supply information about amphetamines.
12. Demonstrate an understanding of hallucinogenic drugs such as LSD, PCP, and mescaline.
13. Demonstrate an understanding of barbiturates.
14. Demonstrate an understanding of the drugs used in dentistry and the ways in which they are used.

SUMMARY

At no other time have drugs been so widely used/misused as they are today. The dental assistant will need to pay attention to the medical and dental history and carefully document the drugs used by the patient. The dental assistant will have to become knowledgeable about pharmacology, the side effects of drugs, and the interactions that take place when more than one drug is used. Dental assistants are concerned with the drugs that are prescribed, but they must have knowledge about illegal drugs that patients may be involved in and what will happen if the two types of drugs interact. It is also important to know the signs and symptoms that individuals may experience if under the influence of drugs. Background knowledge about drugs and their effects aids the dental assistant in providing better patient care.

KEY TERMS

addiction
analgesic
anesthesia
brand names
broad spectrum
closing
Comprehensive Drug Abuse Prevention and Control Act of 1970
Council on Dental Therapeutics
drug

Drug Enforcement Agency (DEA) number
drug interaction
Food and Drug Administration (FDA)
generic names
habit forming
hallucinate
heading
inhalation
inscription
intradermal

intramuscular
intravenous
medicines
oral
over-the-counter (OTC) drugs
pharmacology
Physician's Desk Reference (PDR)
prescription
psychologically dependent
rectal

side effect
subcutaneous
sublingual
subscription
superscription
The Pure Food and Drug Act
The Pure Food, Drug, and Cosmetic Act
topically
withdrawal

EXERCISES AND ACTIVITIES

1. _____ is the study of all drugs.
   A. Medicine   C. Pharmacology
   B. Addiction   D. Parenteral

2. When a person becomes physically dependent on a drug, that person has a(n) _____
   A. interaction.   C. withdrawal.
   B. addiction.   D. prescription.

3. Drugs that cause psychological dependence are referred to as _____
   A. broad spectrum.
   B. brand name.
   C. drug interaction.
   D. habit forming.

4. _____ gathers information about drugs used in dentistry.
   A. CDC
   B. OSHA
   C. Council on Dental Therapeutics
   D. FDA

5. Dentists can obtain information about drugs from several texts. The most commonly used text in the dental office is the _____
   A. DEA.   C. ADA.
   B. FDA.   D. PDR.

6. A prescription is written in several parts. The _____ includes the dentist's name and degrees, office address, and phone number.
   A. heading   C. closing
   B. DEA   D. Rx body

7. In the _____ of the prescription, the dentist inscribes or writes the name and strength of the drug being prescribed, the dose, and in what form the drug is to be dispensed.
   A. heading   C. closing
   B. DEA   D. Rx body

8. The Latin abbreviation b.i.d. in English means _____
   A. before meals.
   B. daily.
   C. twice a day.
   D. take.

9. What law was enacted to control and regulate the composition, sale, and distribution of drugs? _____
   A. PDR
   B. Comprehensive Drug Abuse
   C. FDA
   D. The Pure Food and Drug Act

10. The federal regulation agency that has control of all food, cosmetics, and drugs sold is the _____
    A. DEA
    B. PDR
    C. FDA
    D. Controlled Substance Act

11. Alcohol is a _____, a drug that slows down body processes.
    A. stimulant   C. depressant
    B. narcotic   D. sedative

12. An illegal drug that contains THC and affects the nervous system is _____
    A. nicotine.   C. heroin.
    B. cocaine.   D. marijuana.

13. _____ is the most addictive of the narcotics.
    A. Cocaine   C. Heroin
    B. Marijuana   D. Caffeine

14. One of the best known narcotic analgesic drugs is _____
    A. codeine.   C. amphetamines.
    B. marijuana. D. morphine.

15. Drugs that relieve pain can be non-narcotic such as _____
    A. codeine.   C. amphetamines.
    B. aspirin.   D. morphine.

16. Antibiotics that are effective against a wide range of bacteria are called _____
    A. broad spectrum.
    B. brand names.
    C. drug interaction.
    D. OTC.

17. Schedule _____ drugs, such as marijuana, heroin, and LSD, have a high potential for abuse.
    A. I   C. III
    B. II   D. IV

18. Schedule _____ drugs, such as cocaine and morphine, have a high potential for abuse and lead to physical and psychological dependence.

    A. I   C. III
    B. II   D. IV

19. Schedule _____ drugs, such as Tylenol III, have a lower potential for abuse and are prescribed routinely in the dental office.

    A. I   C. III
    B. II   D. IV

20. The most common method of taking medications is _____

    A. topically.   C. rectally.
    B. orally.   D. sublingually.

21. One of the drugs used in dentistry is nitrous oxide. This drug can be administered _____

    A. sublingually.   C. orally.
    B. topically.   D. by inhalation.

22. _____ is an antifungal drug used in dentistry to treat candidiasis.

    A. Nystatin   C. Atropine
    B. Anticholinergic D. Erythromycin

As we become more knowledgeable about drugs, we also learn about new drugs and drugs being altered. Match the term with its definition.

Term

23. _____ Drug
24. _____ Medicine
25. _____ Side effect
26. _____ Drug interaction
27. _____ Addicted

Definition

A. An unintended result of a drug
B. One drug changes the effect of another drug
C. Physically dependent on a drug
D. Substance that can change life chemical processes
E. Drugs that are used to treat diseases

A prescription is written in several parts. Match the following parts with their use.

Parts

28. _____ Heading
29. _____ Superscription
30. _____ Rx
31. _____ Closing

Use

A. Where dentist signs and authorizes refills
B. Dentist's name, degrees, office address, phone number
C. Patient's name, phone number, age, gender
D. Also the body of the prescription

Match the administration by its route of injection.

Administration

32. _____ Intravenous
33. _____ Intramuscular
34. _____ Subcutaneous
35. _____ Intradermal

Route of Injection

A. Under the epidermis (top layer of skin)
B. Under the skin above the muscle
C. Directly into the vein
D. Into the muscle

CHAPTER 13

Emergency Management

OBJECTIVES

The student should strive to meet the following objectives and demonstrate an understanding of the facts and principles presented in this chapter:

1. Describe several emergency situations that may take place in the dental office. Explain how dental assistants can be prepared for these possibilities.
2. Describe the ABCs of CPR and demonstrate the skills associated with it.
3. Define the terms and anatomy used in the delivery of CPR. Determine whether the patient is unconscious and demonstrate knowledge of opening the airway and when and how to deliver chest compressions.
4. Identify several causes of airway obstructions in the dental office. Demonstrate the ability to open the airway and to perform the Heimlich maneuver, manual and chest thrusts, and the finger sweep.
5. Identify the causes, signs, and treatments of the emergencies of syncope, asthma, allergic reactions, anaphylactic reaction, hyperventilation, epilepsy, diabetes mellitus, hypoglycemia, angina pectoris, myocardial infarction, congestive heart failure, and the stroke/cerebrovascular accident.
6. Identify several dental emergencies that a patient may have, such as abscessed tooth, alveolitis, avulsed tooth, broken prosthesis, soft tissue injury, broken tooth, and loose crown.

SUMMARY

Even though the number of emergencies is not great in a dental office, the dental assistant must always be observant of the patient and be prepared to deal with emergencies. Emergencies may also happen to the dentist and other dental auxiliaries.

When an emergency arises, the dental team must react with an automatic response. Any hesitation at such a time may cost a life. It is best if a routine is established so everyone can ensure everything is taken care of. The assistant has a vital role in the prevention of emergencies and emergency care. Patient observation at all times assists in the prevention evaluation.

KEY TERMS

abscessed tooth	arteriosclerosis	foreign body airway	petit mal seizure
alkalosis	bronchioles	obstruction (FBAO)	status epilepticus
allergens	cardiopulmonary	gingival hyperplasia	sternum
allergic reactions	resuscitation (CPR)	grand mal seizure	stroke
allergy	cerebral embolism	hemiplegia	sublingually
alveolitis	cerebral hemorrhage	hyperventilation	syncope
anaphylactic shock	cerebral infarction	inhaler	transient ischemic attacks
angina pectoris	congestive heart failure	Jacksonian epilepsy	Trendelenburg position
angioedema	diabetes mellitus	myocardial infarction	unconscious
antibodies	edema	oral hypoglycemics	universal distress signal
antigens	epilepsy	partial seizures	urticaria
antihistamines	erythema		

EXERCISES AND ACTIVITIES

1. Which of the following is not a part of the assistant's role in observing the patient for emergency management _____
   A. Is the patient having difficulty moving?
   B. Do the patient's eyes respond to light?
   C. Is the patient's speech slurred?
   D. Does the patient need an injection of epinephrine?
   E. Does the patient indicate anxiety about the dental treatment?

2. Having a well-defined emergency plan will provide the best treatment for the patient. Which of the following is not part of an emergency plan? _____
   A. Everyone knowing the emergency kit location
   B. Everyone knowing the oxygen location
   C. Who will perform CPR
   D. Who will call for help
   E. Who will reschedule patient's next dental appointment

3. The oxygen tank, which is used as a piece of the inhalation equipment, is designated by what color? _____
   A. Blue   C. Green
   B. White   D. Orange

4. If the patient reaches an unconscious state and progresses to a sudden cardiac arrest, what will the first step be? _____
   A. Start CPR.
   B. Phone for help.
   C. Perform the Heimlich.
   D. Remove any artificial appliances.

5. After determining that the patient is unconscious, you have called for help. What is the next step? _____
   A. Look for the chest to rise.
   B. Listen for air exchange.
   C. Feel for any breath.
   D. Tilt the head and lift the chin.

6. Once the airway is open, the rescuer will place his or her ear and face close to the adult patient and _____
   A. look for the chest to rise.
   B. listen for air exchange.
   C. feel for any breath.
   D. All of the above

7. The rescuer administers two slow breaths of how many seconds each for an adult? _____
   A. one and a half to two seconds
   B. one to one and a half seconds
   C. five seconds
   D. three seconds

8. During an adult CPR, the _____ pulse is checked during compression cycles.
   A. brachial   C. carotid
   B. femoral   D. radial

9. If the patient does not have a pulse, an adult would receive compressions at a rate of _____
   A. 100 to 110 per minute.
   B. 80 to 100 per minute.
   C. 90 to 100 per minute.
   D. 80 to 90 per minute.

10. The heels of the rescuer's hand are placed on the _____ of the sternum and compressions begin.
    A. lower third
    B. middle third
    C. upper third
    D. end

11. After every fifteen compressions, deliver _____ more slow breath(s).
    A. four   C. one
    B. two   D. five

12. Repeating the four cycles of compressions and breaths, you will then recheck _____.
    A. hand position
    B. pulse
    C. head tilt
    D. chin lift

13. The electrodes for the defibrillation are placed only if the patient _____
    A. is unconscious.
    B. is not breathing.
    C. has no pulse.
    D. All of the above

14. In the dental office, incidents of _____ are greater than other possible emergencies.
    A. airway obstruction
    B. asthma attacks
    C. partial seizures
    D. cerebral hemorrhage

15. The universal distress signal for an airway obstruction is _____
   A. syncope.
   B. clutching the throat.
   C. convulsing.
   D. clutching the chest.

16. An incident called _____ is when a foreign object lodges into the airway.
   A. Heimlich
   B. CRP
   C. FABO
   D. anaphylactic

17. During an airway obstruction, the patient becomes unconscious. You lay the patient on the floor. Which of the following will be the next critical step? _____
   A. Remove the foreign body.
   B. Activate emergency medical service.
   C. Attempt to give patient breaths.
   D. Reposition head and chin.

18. The most common and least life-threatening emergency that may occur in the dental office is _____
   A. allergic reaction.
   B. anaphylactic shock.
   C. syncope.
   D. angina pectoris.

19. In the dental office, a vasodepressor syncope occurred. This incident is also known as _____
   A. allergic reaction.
   B. anaphylactic shock.
   C. fainting.
   D. seizure.

20. A patient unable to respond to any sensory stimulation is defined as _____
   A. allergic.
   B. urticaria.
   C. hyperplasia.
   D. unconscious.

21. Symptoms of syncope may include _____
   A. dizziness.
   B. nausea.
   C. a feeling of weakness.
   D. All of the above

22. A supine position with the feet elevated above the chest level is called _____
   A. FBAO.
   B. Trendelenburg.
   C. Jacksonian.
   D. Sublingual.

23. The wheezing and breathlessness of an asthma patient is due to the small airways in the _____ narrowing.
   A. antigens
   B. antihistamine
   C. bronchioles
   D. erythemia

24. _____ is an acquired, abnormal response to a substance that does not normally cause a reaction.
   A. Alkalosis
   B. Seizure
   C. Type I mellitus
   D. Allergy

25. A severe allergic reaction that is life threatening is _____
   A. hyperventilation.
   B. hypoglycemia.
   C. anaphylactic shock.
   D. congestive heart failure.

26. _____ is the loss of carbon dioxide from the blood, causing alkalosis.
   A. Hyperglycemia
   B. Hyperventilation
   C. Hypoglycemia
   D. Hemiplegia

27. _____ is the more severe form of diabetes mellitus and occurs between the ages of ten and sixteen.
   A. Type I
   B. Type II
   C. Epilepsy
   D. Hypoglycemia

28. _____ is the result of the pancreas not producing sufficient insulin.
   A. A seizure
   B. Hyperventilation
   C. Diabetes
   D. Angina

29. Too little glucose or sugar causes a person to experience _____
   A. hypoglycemia.
   B. hyperglycemia.
   C. seizures.
   D. allergies.

30. _____ is commonly referred to as hardening of the arteries.
   A. Myocardial infarction
   B. Arteriosclerosis
   C. Cerebrovascular accident (CVA)
   D. Congestive heart failure

31. _____ is a condition in which patient symptoms include pain from pressure, swelling, and severe responses to heat.
   A. Avulsed tooth
   B. Abscessed tooth
   C. Broken prosthesis
   D. Soft tissue injury

32. _____ is a condition commonly known as a dry socket.
    A. Avulsed tooth
    B. Abscessed tooth
    C. Alveolitis
    D. Fistula

Asthma may be caused by an allergy to a substance. Match the term with the definition.

Term
33. _____ Allergy
34. _____ Antibodies
35. _____ Antigens
36. _____ Hypersensitivity
37. _____ Allergens

Definition
A. Body overreacts
B. Antigen triggers allergic reaction
C. Also called immunoglobulins
D. Exaggerated reaction of immune system to offending agent
E. Foreign bodies

A number of other allergic reactions may take place in the dental office, including a dermatitis response. Match the condition with its response.

Condition
38. _____ Allergy
39. _____ Edema
40. _____ Erythema
41. _____ Urticaria
42. _____ Angioedema

Response
A. Large urticaria (hives)
B. Hives may occur on the skin surface
C. Acquired, abnormal immune response to substance
D. Swelling
E. Redness

Epilepsy manifests itself in the form of varying types of seizures. Knowing the characteristics of each may help identify when a colleague or patient is having a seizure and how to respond to it. Following is a listing of types of epilepsy and seizure disorders. Match the term with its characteristics.

Disorder
43. _____ Grand mal seizure
44. _____ Petit mal seizure
45. _____ Jacksonian epilepsy
46. _____ Status epilepticus

Characteristics
A. Continuous seizures
B. Person retains consciousness; also known as a simple partial seizure
C. Momentary loss of consciousness; also known as an absence seizure
D. Lasts two to five minutes; most common seizure

Stroke is a leading cause of disability and death for Americans. Match the term with its condition.

Term
47. _____ Cerebral infarction
48. _____ Cerebral embolism
49. _____ Cerebral hemorrhage
50. _____ Hemiplegia
51. _____ Transient ischemic attacks

Condition
A. Rupture of a blood vessel
B. Weakness, numbness, or paralysis on one side
C. Blood clot
D. Stroke-like symptoms that disappear in twenty-four hours
E. Sudden onset caused by blood loss to brain

SKILL COMPETENCY ASSESSMENT

13-1 Administration of Oxygen

Student's Name _____ Date _____

Instructor's Name _____

SKILL   Identification of the oxygen system used—tanks are stored upright and secure and are green. The oxygen inhalation equipment must be readily available for use at all times.

PERFORMANCE OBJECTIVE   The student will follow a routine procedure that meets the guidelines and protocol to locate oxygen equipment and know how to administer oxygen during an emergency. In some instances, the dental assistant may routinely administer oxygen in conjunction with the nitrous oxide gas under the supervision of the dentist.

	Self Evaluation	Student Evaluation	Possible Points	Instructor Evaluation	Comments
Equipment and Supplies					
1. Oxygen tank with gauge at top or gauge in the dental treatment area			2		
2. Oxygen mask and tubing			2		
Competency Steps					
1. Position the patient comfortably in a supine or Trendelenburg position.			2		
2. Explain the procedure to the patient and reassure the patient that everything is being taken care of (if an emergency should occur).			3		
3. Place the oxygen mask over the patient's nose and drape the tubing on either side of the face (adjust to fit secure over the nose).			3		
4. Start the flow of oxygen immediately. It should flow at two to four liters per minute.			3		
5. Instruct the patient to breathe through his or her nose and have the mouth remain closed.			3		
6. Continue to calm the patient by talking softly in reassuring tones.			2		

TOTAL POINTS POSSIBLE   20

TOTAL POINTS POSSIBLE—2nd Attempt   18

TOTAL POINTS EARNED   _____

Points assigned reflect importance of step to meeting objective: Important = 1; Essential = 2; Critical = 3. Students will lose 2 points for repeated attempts. Failure results if any of the critical steps are omitted or performed incorrectly. If using a 100-point scale, determine score by dividing points earned by total points possible and multiplying the results by 100.

SCORE: _____

SKILL COMPETENCY ASSESSMENT

13-2 Treatment of a Patient with Syncope *(corresponds to textbook Procedure 13-7)*

Student's Name _____ Date _____

Instructor's Name _____

SKILL   Dental assistants must be prepared to identify and treat syncope, or fainting. The onset of syncope may be indicated by dizziness, nausea, extreme weakness, and shallow gasps, and is normally caused by emotional and/or physical stress.

PERFORMANCE OBJECTIVE   The student will follow a routine procedure that meets the guidelines and protocol to position the patient in a Trendelenburg position. The dental assistant must be prepared to treat syncope in the dental office, treatment room, and/or while in the dental chair.

	Self Evaluation	Student Evaluation	Possible Points	Instructor Evaluation	Comments
Equipment and Supplies					
1. Oxygen tank with gauge at top or gauge in the dental treatment area.			2		
2. Oxygen mask and tubing			2		
3. Spirits of ammonia			1		
Competency Steps					
1. Position patient in supine or Trendelenburg position (supine with feet elevated). Observe clothing.			2		
2. Establish that the airway is open. Perform head-tilt, chin-lift to open airway.			3		
3. Breathing normally begins spontaneously within the first ten to fifteen seconds.			1		
4. Administer oxygen as a precaution only.			2		
5. If patient has not revived within the first fifteen seconds, remove the oxygen mask (if one was placed) and pass broken ammonia gauze sponge under patient's nose for one to two seconds.			2		
6. The patient will normally respond rapidly to the pungent odor and take a breath of air.			2		
7. Full revival of the patient should occur within a minute or two.			2		
8. If revival of the patient does not occur, follow the guidelines of CPR.			3		
9. Postpone dental treatment and call for patient transportation.			3		

TOTAL POINTS POSSIBLE   25

TOTAL POINTS POSSIBLE—2nd Attempt   23

TOTAL POINTS EARNED   _____

Points assigned reflect importance of step to meeting objective: Important = 1; Essential = 2; Critical = 3. Students will lose 2 points for repeated attempts. Failure results if any of the critical steps are omitted or performed incorrectly. If using a 100-point scale, determine score by dividing points earned by total points possible and multiplying the results by 100.

SCORE: _____

CHAPTER 14

Introduction to Chairside Assisting

OBJECTIVES

The student should strive to meet the following objectives and demonstrate an understanding of the facts and principles presented in this chapter:

1. Describe the design of a dental office, explaining the purpose of each area.
2. Explain basic concepts of chairside assisting.
3. Describe the necessary steps to prepare a patient for treatment.
4. Explain the necessary steps to seat the patient for treatment.
5. Describe the position of the operator and the assistant at chairside.
6. Describe the necessary steps to dismiss the patient after treatment is concluded.
7. Identify the special needs of certain patients.
8. Describe the grasps, positions, and transfer of instruments for a procedure.
9. Define and demonstrate how to maintain the oral cavity and the equipment utilized in treatment of the oral cavity.

SUMMARY

Dental health professionals go to great lengths to ensure patient and employee safety. It is therefore extremely important to understand the dental setting by facility design, employee role responsibility, and specific job description by procedure.

KEY TERMS

activity zones
air compressor
air-water syringe
amalgamator
central vacuum system
classifications of motion
curing light
delivery systems
dental unit
four-handed dentistry
fulcrum
handpieces

high volume evacuation (HVE)
intraoral camera
laboratory
lumbar
mobile carts
modified pen grasp
operating light
palm grasp
palm-thumb grasp
patient records
pen grasp

reception room
reverse palm-thumb grasp
rheostat
saliva ejector
six-handed dentistry
sterilizing area
subsupine position
supine position
treatment rooms
triturates
ultrasonic scaler

EXERCISES AND ACTIVITIES

1. The decor of which of the following rooms should be changed as often as needed to keep the atmosphere friendly and positive for patients as they enter the dental office? _____
    A. Restroom
    B. Dentist's private office
    C. Reception room
    D. Sterilizing area

2. The dental business office may include which of the following? _____
    1. Appointment scheduling
    2. Filing system
    3. Toothbrush center
    4. Computer terminals
    5. Patient records

    A. 1, 2, 3, 5
    B. 1, 2, 3, 4
    C. 1, 3, 4, 5
    D. 1, 2, 4, 5

3. The assistant should arrive early to open the office and prepare for the day's schedule. Which of the following is not a part of opening the office? _____
    A. Turn on the master switches, lights, dental units, vacuum system, and air compressor.
    B. Turn off water supply to manual processing tanks.
    C. Change into appropriate clinical clothing and follow OSHA guidelines.
    D. Turn on the communication systems.

4. This room should be well ventilated because of chemical fumes and exhaust from equipment. _____
    A. Reception area
    B. Business area
    C. Treatment room
    D. Sterilizing room

5. Dental stools for staff should be made available that provide and meet which of the following requirements? _____
    A. Fixed back rest for vertical adjustment
    B. Good support, comfort
    C. Fixed back rest to support lumbar region
    D. Thin seat
    E. Seat covered with sheepskin

Match each classification of motion with its proper definition.

6. _____ Class I
7. _____ Class II
8. _____ Class III
9. _____ Class IV
10. _____ Class V

A. Involves finger, wrist, and elbow movement
B. Involves movement of the entire arm and shoulder
C. Involves only finger movement
D. Involves movement of the arm and twisting of the body
E. Involves movement of the fingers and wrist

11. Characteristics of good assistant positions are _____
    A. good visibility four to six inches above the operator.
    B. front edge of assistant stool even with patient elbow.
    C. assistant's feet touching the floor.
    D. assistant positioned on stool so weight is on outside edge of seat.

12. The special needs patient is defined as a _____
    A. child patient.
    B. senior patient.
    C. pregnant patient.
    D. hearing impaired.
    E. All of the above

Match each grasp with its proper definition.

13. _____ Pen grasp
14. _____ Palm grasp
15. _____ Palm-thumb
16. _____ Thumb to nose
17. _____ Modified pen

A. Used to hold evacuation tip in patient's mouth
B. Lessens operator fatigue
C. Used with surgical pliers
D. Grasped in the same manner as a pen or pencil
E. Used with instruments having straight shank and blade

The one-handed transfer is the most common instrument transfer. Following are the three steps for the instrument transfer. Match each transfer step with its proper description.

18. _____ Approach
19. _____ Retrieval
20. _____ Delivery

A. Rotate hand toward the operator and place instrument into operator's fingers.
B. Lift the instrument from the tray, holding near the non-working end.
C. Extend little finger and close around the handle of the instrument.

21. Maintaining the operating field is a critical skill for the dental assistant to obtain. Which of the following skills are essential to oral evacuation tip placement? _____
   1. The fingers always rest on the occlusal surface.
   2. The evacuator tip is placed approximately one tooth distal to the tooth being worked on.
   3. The bevel of the tip is held parallel to buccal or lingual surface of the teeth.
   4. The bevel of the tip is parallel to the apex surface of the teeth.
   5. The opening should be even with the occlusal surface.
   6. The primary working end should always be placed toward the cheek.

   A. 1, 5, 6
   B. 2, 3, 5
   C. 2, 3, 6
   D. 1, 3, 5

SKILL COMPETENCY ASSESSMENT

▌14-1 Seating the Dental Patient *(corresponds to textbook Procedure 14-3)*

Student's Name _____ Date _____

Instructor's Name _____

SKILL Greet the patient in the reception area and escort the patient to the treatment room. Prepare the patient for the dental treatment.

PERFORMANCE OBJECTIVE The student will review the patient's medical and dental records, clean and prepare the treatment room with appropriate barriers, ready the tray setup, and remove any possible obstacles from the patient's pathway.

	Self Evaluation	Student Evaluation	Possible Points	Instructor Evaluation	Comments
Equipment and Supplies					
1. Patient's medical and dental records			1		
2. Basic setup: mouth mirror, explorer, and cotton pliers			1		
3. Saliva ejector, evacuator (HVE), and air-water syringe tip			1		
4. Cotton rolls, cotton-tip applicator, and gauze sponges			1		
5. Lip lubricant			1		
6. Tissue			1		
7. Protective eyewear			1		
Competency Steps					
1. Greet and escort the patient to the treatment room. Show patient where to place personal items. You may offer mouth rinse.			3		
2. Seat the patient in the dental chair. Have the patient sit all the way back in the chair. Offer patient tissue to remove lipstick and offer lubricant for the lips.			3		
3. Place the bib on the patient and give the patient protective eyewear.			2		
4. Review the patient's health history for any changes since the last visit. Check whether patient has any questions. Provide a brief explanation/confirmation of treatment being completed at this appointment.			3		
5. Position the patient for treatment, adjust the headrest, and adjust the dental light for the appropriate arch.			3		
6. Position the operator's stool and the rheostat.			2		

14-1 continued *(corresponds to textbook Procedure 14-3)*

	Self Evaluation	Student Evaluation	Possible Points	Instructor Evaluation	Comments
7. Position the assistant's stool. Put on mask and protective eyewear, then wash hands and place on gloves before being seated chairside.			3		
8. Position the tray setup. Prepare the saliva ejector, evacuator tip, air-water (three-way) syringe tip, and dental handpieces.			3		

TOTAL POINTS POSSIBLE   29

TOTAL POINTS POSSIBLE—2nd Attempt   27

TOTAL POINTS EARNED   _____

Points assigned reflect importance of step to meeting objective: Important = 1; Essential = 2; Critical = 3. Students will lose 2 points for repeated attempts. Failure results if any of the critical steps are omitted or performed incorrectly. If using a 100-point scale, determine score by dividing points earned by total points possible and multiplying the results by 100.

SCORE: _____

SKILL COMPETENCY ASSESSMENT

14-2 **Dismissing the Dental Patient** *(corresponds to textbook Procedure 14-4)*

Student's Name _____ Date _____

Instructor's Name _____

SKILL After the treatment is completed, the patient is escorted from the treatment room to the reception area.

PERFORMANCE OBJECTIVE The student will remove gloves, wash hands, and review the patient's dental treatment with the dentist. Documentation will be made on the patient's chart or in the computer terminal by the assistant. The patient's chart and x-rays are gathered, the patient's personal items are returned, any obstacles are removed from the patient's pathway, and the patient is escorted to the reception area.

	Self Evaluation	Student Evaluation	Possible Points	Instructor Evaluation	Comments
Equipment and Supplies					
1. Patient's medical and dental records			1		
2. Basic setup: mouth mirror, explorer, and cotton pliers			1		
3. Saliva ejector, evacuator (HVE), and air-water syringe tip			1		
4. Cotton rolls, cotton-tip applicator, and gauze sponges			1		
5. Lip lubricant			1		
6. Tissue			1		
7. Protective eyewear			1		
Competency Steps					
1. When operator is finished with procedure, rinse and evacuate the patient's mouth thoroughly. Patient is placed in an upright position, bib is removed, and patient directed to remain seated. Patient bib is used to cover the tray.			3		
2. Remove any debris from the patient's face. (Patient can also look in mirror before leaving the treatment area.)			2		
3. Remove evacuator (HVE) tip, saliva ejector, air-water syringe tip.			2		
4. Dental light positioned out of the way. Operator's stool and rheostat are moved out of way of patient.			3		
5. Procedure documented in the patient chart or in the computer terminal (gloves must be removed and hands washed). Patient's chart and x-rays gathered.			3		
6. Post-operative instructions given to patient.			2		

14-2 continued *(corresponds to textbook Procedure 14-4)*

	Self Evaluation	Student Evaluation	Possible Points	Instructor Evaluation	Comments
7. Patient's personal items returned and patient is escorted to reception area.			1		

TOTAL POINTS POSSIBLE   23

TOTAL POINTS POSSIBLE—2nd Attempt   21

TOTAL POINTS EARNED   _____

Points assigned reflect importance of step to meeting objective: Important = 1; Essential = 2; Critical = 3. Students will lose 2 points for repeated attempts. Failure results if any of the critical steps are omitted or performed incorrectly. If using a 100-point scale, determine score by dividing points earned by total points possible and multiplying the results by 100.

SCORE: _____

SKILL COMPETENCY ASSESSMENT

14-3 One-Handed Instrument Transfer *(corresponds to textbook Procedure 14-5)*

Student's Name _____ Date _____

Instructor's Name _____

SKILL The one-handed transfer is the most common transfer. The assistant picks up the next instrument to be transferred with one hand and with the same hand receives the instrument the operator is finished using, and then rotates the new instrument into the operator's hand.

PERFORMANCE OBJECTIVE The student will demonstrate the exchange of dental instruments in a safe and efficient manner with the working end delivered in the position of use.

	Self Evaluation	Student Evaluation	Possible Points	Instructor Evaluation	Comments
Equipment and Supplies					
1. Basic setup: mouth mirror, explorer, and cotton pliers			3		
2. Spoon excavator (for pen or modified pen grasp)			2		
3. Straight chisel, forceps, or elevators (for palm grasp)			2		
Competency Steps					
Approach					
1. Lift instrument from tray, using thumb, index finger, and second finger. Hold the instrument near non-working end.			3		
2. Turn palm upward into passing position, rotating nib toward correct arch.			3		
3. Move toward operator's hand.			2		
Retrieval					
4. Extend little finger and close around handle of instrument the operator is holding.			3		
5. Lift instrument out of the operator's hand.			3		
6. Pull this instrument toward assistant's palm and wrist.			3		
Delivery					
7. Rotate hand toward operator and place instrument in operator's fingers.			3		

14-3 continued *(corresponds to textbook Procedure 14-5)*

	Self Evaluation	Student Evaluation	Possible Points	Instructor Evaluation	Comments
8. Once operator has new instrument, rotate it to delivery position for use again or return it to tray.			3		

TOTAL POINTS POSSIBLE   30

TOTAL POINTS POSSIBLE—2nd Attempt   28

TOTAL POINTS EARNED   _____

Points assigned reflect importance of step to meeting objective: Important = 1; Essential = 2; Critical = 3. Students will lose 2 points for repeated attempts. Failure results if any of the critical steps are omitted or performed incorrectly. If using a 100-point scale, determine score by dividing points earned by total points possible and multiplying the results by 100.

SCORE: _____

SKILL COMPETENCY ASSESSMENT

14-4 Specific Tip Placements for Evacuation of the Oral Cavity
(corresponds to textbook Procedure 14-6)

Student's Name _____ Date _____

Instructor's Name _____

SKILL   To maintain the oral cavity to keep the area clear and clean for the operator and for comfort of the patient.

PERFORMANCE OBJECTIVE   The student will demonstrate the various oral evacuation tip placements for each quadrant when assisting a right-handed operator.

	Self Evaluation	Student Evaluation	Possible Points	Instructor Evaluation	Comments
Equipment and Supplies					
1. Basic setup: mouth mirror, cotton pliers, and explorer			1		
2. HVE tip and air-water syringe tip			1		
3. Cotton rolls			1		
Competency Steps					
1. Carefully place the evacuator tip into the patient's mouth (avoiding bumping the teeth, lips, or gingiva).			3		
2. Evacuator tip is placed into the mouth and positioned before the operator positions the handpiece or instrument.			2		
3. The evacuation tip is placed approximately one tooth distal to the tooth being worked on.			2		
4. The bevel of the evacuator tip is held parallel to assigned surface (buccal or lingual).			2		
5. The middle of the evacuator tip opening is even with the occlusal surface.			1		
6. The evacuator tip is held still while the handpiece or instruments are being used or exchanged.			2		
7. Evacuator tip is not resting on gingival tissue.			3		
8. Demonstrate areas of the mouth to avoid so as to not gag the patient.			2		
9. The evacuator tip is kept away from the mucosal tissue.			2		

TOTAL POINTS POSSIBLE   22

TOTAL POINTS POSSIBLE—2nd Attempt   20

TOTAL POINTS EARNED   _____

Points assigned reflect importance of step to meeting objective: Important = 1; Essential = 2; Critical = 3. Students will lose 2 points for repeated attempts. Failure results if any of the critical steps are omitted or performed incorrectly. If using a 100-point scale, determine score by dividing points earned by total points possible and multiplying the results by 100.

SCORE: _____

Chairside Instruments and Tray Systems

OBJECTIVES

The student should strive to meet the following objectives and demonstrate an understanding of the facts and principles presented in this chapter:

1. Identify the parts of an instrument and describe how instruments are identified.
2. Identify the categories and functions of dental burs.
3. Describe the types and functions of abrasives.
4. Explain the various handpieces and attachments.
5. Describe the types of tray systems and color-coding systems.

SUMMARY

The basic instruments used in general dental procedures include common cutting and non-cutting instruments. Instruments are generally categorized into hand instruments and rotary instruments. Each procedure has special instruments to accomplish specific tasks. It is the assistant's responsibility to keep the instruments sterilized, organized, and in working condition.

KEY TERMS

abrasives
air abrasion
bevel
binangle
Black's formula
blade
burs
chuck

contra-angle
cutting edge
fiberoptic light sources
frictional heat
high-speed handpieces
low-speed handpieces
mandrels
manufacturer's number

monangle
non-cutting
revolutions per minute
    (rpm)
rotary instruments
shaft
shank
working end

EXERCISES AND ACTIVITIES

1. Which of the following is not a part of the dental hand instrument? _____
   A. Flute
   B. Handle
   C. Shank
   D. Working end

2. The _____ is the part of the instrument that connects the handle to the working end.
   A. handle
   B. shank
   C. blade
   D. bevel

3. The working end of the instrument may be a _____
   A. point.
   B. blade.
   C. nib.
   D. All of the above

4. Which part of the instrument actually performs the specific function of the instrument? _____
   A. Handle
   B. Shank
   C. Working end
   D. Flute

5. _____ formula was developed to standardize the exact size and angulation of an instrument.
   A. Manufacturer's number
   B. Black's
   C. First number
   D. Second number

6. Which of the following is not a cutting instrument? _____
   A. Chisel
   B. Excavator
   C. Carrier
   D. Angle former

7. Which of the following is not a non-cutting instrument? _____
   A. Carver
   B. Carrier
   C. File
   D. Hoe

8. Which of the following is not a part of Black's three-number formula? _____
   A. The first number is the width of the blade.
   B. The second number is the measurement of the length of the blade.
   C. The second number represents the degree of angle of the cutting edge to the blade.
   D. The third number gives the measurement of the angle of the blade to the long axis of the handle.

9. _____ are used to assist in the design of the cavity preparation.
   A. Amalgam carriers
   B. Carvers
   C. Amalgam condensers
   D. Hand cutting instruments

10. _____ are used to shape and plane enamel and dentin walls of the cavity preparation.
    A. Hoes
    B. Hatchets
    C. Chisels
    D. Angle formers
    E. Gingival margin trimmers

11. _____ are paired left and right and are used in a downward motion to refine the cavity walls.
    A. Excavators
    B. Hatchets
    C. Hoes
    D. Chisels

12. The _____ is used in a pulling motion to smooth and shape the floor of the cavity preparation.
    A. gingival margin trimmer
    B. hatchet
    C. hoe
    D. chisel

13. The _____ is similar to the hatchet in regard to the position of the blade to the handle and is used to bevel the gingival margin wall of the cavity preparation.
    A. hatchet
    B. gingival margin trimmer
    C. hoe
    D. chisel

14. The _____ is used in a downward pushing motion to form and define point angles and to sharpen line angles.
    A. gingival margin trimmer
    B. angle former
    C. hatchet
    D. chisel

15. The _____, used to remove carious material, has a cutting edge that is rounded all the way around the periphery of the blade.
    A. gingival margin trimmer
    B. carrier
    C. excavator
    D. carver

16. The _____ examination setup instruments are common to all tray setups.
    A. composite
    B. plastic
    C. basic
    D. amalgam

17. Which of the following is not a part of the basic examination setup instruments? _____
    A. Excavator
    B. Mouth mirror
    C. Explorer
    D. Cotton pliers

18. Which is not a type of mouth mirror? _____
    A. Concave   C. Front
    B. Convex   D. Plane

19. When the operator uses a mirror to view areas of the mouth not visible with direct vision, this is called _____
    A. retraction of light.
    B. transillumination.
    C. indirect vision.
    D. direct vision.

20. When the mirror is used to direct the light to reflect and detect fractures in a tooth, this is called _____
    A. retraction.
    B. transillumination.
    C. indirect vision.
    D. direct vision.

21. Which instrument's working end is a thin, sharp point of flexible steel? _____
    A. Excavator
    B. Cotton pliers
    C. Explorer
    D. Plastic instrument

22. _____ are used to transport and manipulate various materials. They are available in locking or non-locking handles.
    A. Explorers
    B. Excavators
    C. Cotton pliers
    D. Probes

23. The working end of the _____ is a blade that is rounded or blunted and is marked in millimeters.
    A. explorer   C. plastic
    B. probe   D. carver

24. The amalgam _____ is designed to carry and dispense amalgam into the cavity preparation.
    A. condenser   C. carver
    B. carrier   D. burnisher

25. _____ are used to remove excess restorative material and carve tooth anatomy in the restoration before the material hardens.
    A. Condensers   C. Carvers
    B. Carriers   D. Burnishers

26. _____ knives are used to trim excess filling material.
    A. Carver   C. File
    B. Finishing   D. Burnisher

27. _____ spatulas are used to mix composite resin materials.
    A. Cement   C. Plastic
    B. Laboratory   D. Surgical

28. Which of the following is not a use or characteristic of the crown and collar scissors? _____
    A. Trim matrix bands
    B. Cut retraction cord
    C. Trim amalgam
    D. Straight blade

29. The _____ of the bur is inserted into the handpiece.
    A. neck   C. diamond
    B. head   D. shank

30. The _____ of the bur is the working end of the bur.
    A. neck   C. diamond
    B. head   D. shank

31. Cutting burs have _____ cutting blades or surfaces.
    A. six   C. twelve
    B. four   D. ten

32. There are _____ basic cutting bur shapes.
    A. three   C. nine
    B. six   D. twelve

33. _____ burs or stones are used for rapid reduction of tooth structure during cavity preparation, polishing and finishing composite restorations, and occlusal adjustment.
    A. Surgical   C. Laboratory
    B. Finishing   D. Diamond

34. _____ are non-bladed instruments used to finish and polish restorations.
    A. Abrasives   C. Mandrels
    B. Diamonds   D. Finishing burs

35. Which of the following instruments have abrasive material that may be made of garnet, diamond, and quartz? _____
    A. Cutting burs
    B. Fissure burs
    C. Discs
    D. Finishing burs

36. _____ discs are used for rapid cutting and have diamond particles bonded to both sides of steel discs.
    A. Sandpaper   C. Carborundum
    B. Diamond   D. Separating

37. The _____ end of the handpiece is where burs, stones, and attachments are held.
    A. connection   C. rheostat
    B. working   D. shank

38. Which of the following will reduce frictional heat from the use of the high speed? _____
    A. Air
    B. Water
    C. Air-water spray
    D. All of the above

39. The _____ holds the shank portion of the bur in place.
    A. head   C. handle
    B. chuck   D. neck

40. What will activate and control the speed of the handpiece? _____
    A. Power source
    B. Fiberoptic light source
    C. Friction
    D. Rheostat

41. The low-speed handpiece is often referred to as the _____
    A. Contra-angle.
    B. Right-angle.
    C. straight handpiece.
    D. latch type.

42. At the dental unit, the low-speed handpiece will not _____
    A. polish teeth.
    B. remove soft carious material.
    C. polish appliances.
    D. define cavity walls.

43. Which of the following cannot be sterilized? _____
    A. Burs
    B. Handpieces
    C. Sandpaper discs
    D. Rotary instruments

44. High-speed handpieces operate at _____
    A. 400,000 rpm.
    B. 30,000 rpm.
    C. 100,000 rpm.
    D. 250,000 rpm.

45. A _____ tray system provides an efficient means to transport instruments.
    A. positioning   C. rubberized
    B. preset   D. color-coded

46. The _____ chisel is used for Class III or IV cavity preparation.
    A. straight   C. Wedelstaedt
    B. binangle   D. contra-angle

47. Which of the following is not a use of the dental handpiece? _____
    A. To remove dental decay
    B. To polish teeth
    C. To polish and finish restorations
    D. To probe

Hand cutting instruments are used to assist in the design of the cavity preparation. Match the instrument with its use.

Instrument
48. _____ Hatchet
49. _____ Hoe
50. _____ Gingival margin trimmer
51. _____ Angle former
52. _____ Chisel

Use
A. Used in pulling motion to shape floor of cavity preparation
B. Shape and plane enamel/dentin walls of cavity preparation
C. Used in downward motion to form/define point angles
D. Bevel gingival margin wall of cavity preparation
E. Used in downward motion to refine cavity walls

Instruments are classified by function to describe the specific use. Match the non-cutting instrument with its use.

Instrument

53. _____ Amalgam carriers
54. _____ Amalgam gun
55. _____ Amalgam condensers
56. _____ Carvers
57. _____ Burnishers

Use

A. Sometimes called pluggers
B. Carry and dispense into cavity preparation
C. Carve tooth anatomy in restoration
D. Smooth rough margins
E. Has spring action and is single-ended and made of plastic

Dental burs are a part of a group of instruments referred to as rotary instruments. Match the part of the bur with its description.

Bur

58. _____ Shank
59. _____ Neck
60. _____ Head

Description

A. Working end of the bur
B. Inserted into the handpiece
C. Tapered connection of the shank to the head

Identify the bur name with its function.

Bur Name

61. _____ Round
62. _____ Inverted cone
63. _____ Plain fissure straight
64. _____ Tapered fissure cross-cut
65. _____ Diamond

Function

A. Forms cavity walls of preparation
B. Used for rapid reduction of tooth structure
C. Used to open the cavity and remove caries
D. Makes undercuts and removes caries
E. Forms divergent walls of the cavity preparation

66. Most instruments are constructed of stainless steel.

A. True
B. False

Management of Pain and Anxiety

The student should strive to meet the following objectives and demonstrate an understanding of the facts and principles presented in this chapter:

1. Describe methods used to manage the pain and anxiety related to dental procedures.
2. Explain different types of topical anesthetics and their placements.
3. Describe types of local anesthetics.
4. List the steps for preparing for the administration of local anesthetic.
5. Identify the injection sites for the maxillary and mandibular arches.
6. Describe the equipment and materials needed to administer local anesthetic.
7. Identify supplemental techniques to administer anesthetics.
8. Discuss the role of nitrous oxide in the care of the dental patient.
9. Demonstrate the ability to assist in the administration of nitrous oxide.

SUMMARY

Because most procedures require some form of anesthesia, the dentist may select one or a combination of methods to control pain, depending on the patient and the procedure to be completed. The dental assistant is responsible for preparing, safely transferring, and caring for the anesthetic syringe and accessories. During this time, the assistant must be aware of the various topical solutions, application sites, how to apply the topical anesthetic, and possible patient reactions. In addition, the assistant follows the dentist's directions for the administration of sedation and monitoring requirements.

KEY TERMS

carpules	field block anesthesia	nerve block anesthesia
cartridges	general anesthetic	nitrous oxide
computer-controlled local anesthesia	infiltration anesthesia	topical anesthetic
	local anesthesia	vasoconstrictors

EXERCISES AND ACTIVITIES

1. When a(n) _____ anesthetic is administered, the patient becomes unconscious.
   - A. local
   - B. topical
   - C. general
   - D. infiltration

2. _____ anesthesia produces a deadened or pain-free area.
   - A. Sedation
   - B. General
   - C. Topical
   - D. Local

3. _____ anesthetics desensitize the oral mucosa.
   - A. Local
   - B. Topical
   - C. General
   - D. Infiltration

4. The _____ reaction is a hypersensitive reaction to anesthetic solution.
   - A. toxic
   - B. paresthesia
   - C. allergic
   - D. intraosseous

5. The _____ reactions are symptoms due to an overdose or excessive administration of anesthetic solution.
   - A. allergic
   - B. toxic
   - C. paresthesia
   - D. topical

6. Local anesthetics used for injections are available in _____ form.
   - A. topical
   - B. gas
   - C. liquid
   - D. gel

7. Which of the following is not an amide compound found in local anesthetic solutions? _____
   - A. Lidocaine
   - B. Mepivacaine
   - C. Prilocaine
   - D. Procaine

8. _____ duration solutions will last longer than ninety minutes and contain a vasoconstrictor.
   - A. Intermediate
   - B. Long
   - C. Short
   - D. All of the above

9. The most common vasoconstrictor used in dentistry is _____
   - A. oxygen.
   - B. nitrous oxide sedation.
   - C. epinephrine.
   - D. distilled water.

10. Which of the following is not among the most common vasoconstrictor ratios? _____
    - A. 1:20,000
    - B. 1:50,000
    - C. 1:10,000
    - D. 1:100,000

11. _____ is the sensation of feeling numb.
    - A. Hemorrhage
    - B. Paresthesia
    - C. Impulse
    - D. Allergic

12. The injection method that places anesthetic solution into tissue near the small terminal nerve branches for absorption is _____
    - A. computer.
    - B. local.
    - C. field block.
    - D. nerve block.

13. The injection method that deposits anesthetic near larger terminal nerve branches is _____
    - A. nerve block.
    - B. computer.
    - C. local.
    - D. field block.

14. The injection method that deposits anesthetic solutions near a main nerve trunk is _____
    - A. field block.
    - B. computer.
    - C. electronic.
    - D. nerve block.

15. The _____ part of the syringe is cleaned with a brush and checked for sharpness prior to sterilizing.
    - A. barrel
    - B. piston rod
    - C. threaded end
    - D. harpoon

16. Which injection would use a long needle? _____
    - A. Infiltration
    - B. Incisive
    - C. Mental
    - D. Infraorbital

17. The internal opening of the needle, where the anesthetic solution flows through, is called the _____
    - A. hub.
    - B. shank.
    - C. lumen.
    - D. harpoon.

18. The _____ is the slanted tip of the needle.
    - A. lumen
    - B. gauge
    - C. bevel
    - D. shank

19. The part of the needle that attaches to the threaded end of the syringe is the _____
    - A. shank.
    - B. hub.
    - C. syringe end.
    - D. harpoon.

20. This cylinder contains the anesthetic solution. _____
    A. Computer   C. Electronic
    B. Cartridge   D. Topical

21. The _____ is where the syringe end of the needle penetrates into the anesthetic solution.
    A. aluminum cap
    B. rubber plunger
    C. piston rod
    D. diaphragm

22. Which of the following conditions would indicate the anesthetic cartridge should be discarded? _____
    A. Large bubbles
    B. Extruded plunger
    C. Corrosion
    D. All of the above

23. The injection that places local anesthetic directly into the cancellous bone is _____
    A. periodontal ligament.
    B. intrapulpal.
    C. electronic.
    D. intraosseous.

24. Benefits from use of nitrous oxide sedation include which of the following? _____
    A. Provides relaxation and relieves apprehension
    B. Makes time pass quickly
    C. Allows patient to be comfortable while receiving treatment
    D. All of the above

25. Which of the following is a contraindication for the use of nitrous oxide sedation? _____
    A. Patients unable to breathe through their noses
    B. Patients who are fearful of dental treatment
    C. Patients who have a gag reflex that is very sensitive
    D. Patients who have a heart condition and will benefit because of oxygen

26. The _____ meter adjusts the gas flow through the unit.
    A. reservoir   C. nosepiece
    B. flow   D. mask

27. The nitrous oxide gas cylinder color is _____
    A. white.   C. green.
    B. blue.   D. orange.

28. The concentration of solution for a topical anesthetic is _____ than the concentration of solution used for local anesthetics.
    A. higher   B. lower

29. The _____ needle is used for injections that require little penetration of the soft tissue such as infiltration.
    A. long   B. short

30. The _____ needle is used for mandibular nerve block injections.
    A. short   B. long

31. Nitrous oxide sedation will _____ the pain threshold without the loss of consciousness.
    A. lower   B. raise

Following are injection sites. Match the injection with the teeth most affected.

Injection
32. _____ Infiltration
33. _____ Middle superior alveolar
34. _____ Inferior alveolar nerve
35. _____ Mental nerve block

Effect
A. A mandibular quadrant
B. Mandibular premolars, canines
C. Maxillary premolars in one quadrant
D. Individual teeth

The type of syringe most commonly used for dental procedures is the aspirating syringe. Recommended by the ADA, it is designed to allow the operator to check the position of the needle before depositing the anesthetic solution. Match the part with its function.

Part
36. _____ Thumb ring
37. _____ Plunger
38. _____ Harpoon
39. _____ Threaded end
40. _____ Barrel

Function
A. Holds the cartridge
B. Barbed tip end that engages cartridge
C. Where needle attaches to syringe
D. Allows operator to aspirate; should not come loose
E. Located inside the syringe; the rod applies force

SKILL COMPETENCY ASSESSMENT

16-1 Preparing the Anesthetic Syringe

Student's Name _____ Date _____

Instructor's Name _____

SKILL   Routine steps should be followed for all patients in the management of pain and anxiety. The dental assistant must be aware of the various anesthetic solutions, techniques, application sites, and possible patient reactions.

PERFORMANCE OBJECTIVE   The student will follow a routine procedure that meets the regulations and the protocol set forth by the dentist and regulatory agencies, keeping in mind that assistants' duties vary from state to state. The dental assistant prepares the syringe out of the view of the patient (the dentist places the topical or if the dental assistant is an expanded functions dental assistant, the assistant places the topical anesthetic and then loads the syringe).

	Self Evaluation	Student Evaluation	Possible Points	Instructor Evaluation	Comments
Equipment and Supplies					
1. Sterile syringe			2		
2. Selected disposable needle			2		
3. Selected anesthetic cartridge			3		
4. 2 x 2 gauze sponge moistened with 91 percent isopropyl alcohol or 70 percent ethyl alcohol			1		
Competency Steps					
1. Following aseptic procedures, select disposable needle and anesthetic the dentist has specified for this procedure (right-handed op).			3		
2. Remove the sterile syringe from autoclave bag. Inspect syringe to be sure it is ready for use.			2		
3. Hold syringe in left hand and use thumb ring to retract piston rod fully.			3		
4. With piston rod retracted, place cartridge in barrel of syringe. Once cartridge is in place, release the piston rod (rubber stopper toward piston).			3		
5. With moderate pressure, push the piston rod into the rubber stopper until it is fully engaged.			3		
6. Remove the protective plastic cap from the syringe end of the needle, and then screw or press needle onto syringe hub. Needle must be secure but not too tight. Needle guards are often placed on protective cap.			3		

16-1 continued

	Self Evaluation	Student Evaluation	Possible Points	Instructor Evaluation	Comments
7. Carefully remove protective cover from the needle. Holding syringe, expel a few drops to ensure syringe is properly working.			3		

TOTAL POINTS POSSIBLE	28
TOTAL POINTS POSSIBLE—2nd Attempt	26
TOTAL POINTS EARNED	_____

Points assigned reflect importance of step to meeting objective: Important = 1; Essential = 2; Critical = 3. Students will lose 2 points for repeated attempts. Failure results if any of the critical steps are omitted or performed incorrectly. If using a 100-point scale, determine score by dividing points earned by total points possible and multiplying the results by 100.

SCORE: _____

SKILL COMPETENCY ASSESSMENT

16-2 Assisting with the Administration of Topical and Local Anesthetics

Student's Name _____ Date _____

Instructor's Name _____

SKILL   The dental assistant will observe safety precautions at all times during this procedure. The patient is informed on the procedure but not alerted to words such as "pain," "shot," and so on.

PERFORMANCE OBJECTIVE   The student will follow a routine procedure that meets the regulations and the protocol set forth by the dentist and regulatory agencies, keeping in mind that assistants' duties vary from state to state. The dental assistant checks with the dentist for instructions on the type of anesthetic and needle for the procedure. Following those instructions, the assistant will prepare the equipment and material on the procedure tray setup.

	Self Evaluation	Student Evaluation	Possible Points	Instructor Evaluation	Comments
Equipment and Supplies					
1. Patient's medical dental history and chart			2		
2. Basic setup: mouth mirror, explorer, and cotton pliers			2		
3. Air-water syringe tip and evacuator tip (HVE)			2		
4. Cotton rolls, cotton-tip applicator, and 2 x 2 gauze sponges			2		
5. Topical anesthetic			1		
6. Aspirating syringe			2		
7. Anesthetic cartridge			2		
8. Selection of needles			2		
Competency Steps					
Topical Anesthetic					
1. After seating patient, review and update the medical dental history.			2		
2. Explain the procedure and prepare patient for topical application.			2		
3. Follow aseptic procedures; place small amount of topical anesthetic on cotton-tip applicator.			1		
4. Dry oral mucosa with sterile 2 x 2 gauze sponge. Keep tissue retracted.			2		
5. Place topical anesthetic on injection site and leave for one minute.			3		
Local Anesthetic					
6. While waiting for topical, assemble the syringe, cartridge, and needle as prescribed by dentist.			3		
7. When operator indicates, take the cotton-tip applicator and prepare to pass the syringe.			2		

16-2 continued

	Self Evaluation	Student Evaluation	Possible Points	Instructor Evaluation	Comments
8. Check the needle bevel so it is directed toward the alveolar bone, and then loosely replace the cap on the needle.			3		
9. Pass the syringe below the patient's chin, placing the thumb ring over the dentist's thumb. Once the dentist grasps the syringe at the finger rest and takes the syringe, remove the protective guard.			3		
10. The injection is completed and the operator recaps the syringe by sliding the needle into the protective guard. If a second injection is given, remove the cartridge, insert a new one, test syringe by expelling a few drops, check bevel, and position the needle for the dentist to retrieve.			3		
11. The recapped syringe is placed on tray, out of the way but near in case more anesthetic is needed.			2		
12. Rinse the patient's mouth with air-water syringe and evacuate to remove water, saliva, and taste of anesthetic solution.			2		
Unloading the Anesthetic Syringe					
1. After procedure is completed and the patient is dismissed, put on utility gloves to clean up, take apart the syringe, and prepare it for sterilization.			2		
2. Carefully remove the needle with protective cap in place. Carefully unscrew needle (do not unscrew needle adapter). Needle is discarded into sharps.			3		
3. Retract piston to release harpoon from cartridge.			2		
4. Remove cartridge from syringe.			2		
5. Prepare syringe for sterilization.			2		

TOTAL POINTS POSSIBLE   54

TOTAL POINTS POSSIBLE—2nd Attempt   52

TOTAL POINTS EARNED   _____

Points assigned reflect importance of step to meeting objective: Important = 1; Essential = 2; Critical = 3. Students will lose 2 points for repeated attempts. Failure results if any of the critical steps are omitted or performed incorrectly. If using a 100-point scale, determine score by dividing points earned by total points possible and multiplying the results by 100.

SCORE: _____

Dental Radiography

OBJECTIVES

The student should strive to meet the following objectives and demonstrate an understanding of the facts and principles presented in this chapter:

1. Explain the history of radiation and the use of the Hittorf-Crookes and Coolidge tubes.
2. List the properties of radiation and explain the biological effects of radiation exposure.
3. Identify the components of a dental x-ray unit and explain the function of each component.
4. Describe the safety precautions to be utilized when using radiation.
5. Explain how an x-ray is produced.
6. Describe the composition, sizes, types, and storage of dental x-ray film.
7. Explain intraoral and extraoral x-ray production.
8. Identify means of producing quality radiographs on a variety of patients.
9. Explain the bisecting and paralleling techniques.
10. List common production errors.
11. Describe the processing techniques, the composition of the solutions, and the storage of final radiographs.
12. Explain the mounting procedures.
13. Identify extraoral films and describe exposing techniques.
14. Identify normal and abnormal radiographic landmarks.
15. List standardized procedures and state policies that dental offices follow to ensure quality radiographs.
16. Identify imaging systems used for dental purposes.

SUMMARY

It is the responsibility of the manufacturers, dental team members, and patients to follow safety and precaution measures when using radiography equipment. Steps must be used to minimize risk to the patient and all dental personnel.

The dentist is responsible for having dental assistants properly credentialed and trained to expose and process radiographs. The dentist is also responsible for supervising dental assistants in these tasks. In 1981, the Consumer Patient Radiation Health and Safety Act was enacted. This federal law requires each state to inform the Secretary of Health and Human Services how compliance with the act is accomplished.

The dental assistant must be trained in aseptic techniques, radiation hygiene, and maintenance of quality assurance and safety and must obtain a proper education in exposure and processing techniques. He or she must have an understanding of the physics and biological effects of ionizing radiation and utilize the understanding during every radiographic exposure and must understand the ALARA principle and utilize the lead apron with cervical collar for the patient's safety each time an x-ray is taken. The assistant must label and store patient x-rays properly to prevent loss and thus the need for x-rays being retaken.

KEY TERMS

ALARA
anode
automatic processing
basal cells
bisecting technique
bitewing
blurred images
cassette
cathode
central beam
cephalometric radiographs
collimator
computed tomography
    (CT scanning)
cone cutting
cross-section technique
developer solution
digital imaging technology
double exposure
duplication technique
electromagnetic energy
elongation
extraoral film
fixer solution

focal spot
focusing cup
foreshortening
Frankfort plane
Gray (GY)
herringbone pattern
horizontal angulation
intensifying screens
interproximal
intraoral
kilovoltage (kV)
latent period
leakage radiation
long wavelengths
magnetic resonance imaging (MRI)
manual processing
maximum permissible dose (MPD)
milliamperage (mA)
milliroentgen (mr)
mitosis
occlusal radiographs
overlapping
panoramic technique
paralleling technique

periapical
primary radiation
radiation absorbed dose (rad)
radiolucent
radiopaque
radiosensitive
relative biological effectiveness
    (rbe)
reticulation
roentgens
roentgen equivalent man (rem)
scatter radiation
secondary radiation
short wavelengths
sievert (Sv)
targus of the ear
thermionic emission
topographic technique
transcranial temporomandibular
    joint radiograph
tubehead
vertical angulation
x-ray tube
x-rays

EXERCISES AND ACTIVITIES

1. _____ was a professor of physics and discovered x-rays.
   A. Kells
   B. Roentgen
   C. Walkoff
   D. Rollins

2. _____ took the first intraoral radiograph.
   A. Walkoff
   B. Roentgen
   C. Kells
   D. Rollins

3. _____ developed the bisecting technique.
   A. Rober
   B. McCormack
   C. Fitzgerald
   D. Coolidge

4. _____ developed the paralleling technique.
   A. Fitzgerald
   B. Coolidge
   C. Rober
   D. McCormack

5. The open-ended tube, commonly referred to as the cone, is called the _____
   A. position indicator device (PID).
   B. maximum permissible dose (MPD).
   C. radiation absorbed dose (rad).
   D. roentgen equivalent man (rem).

6. Other forms of electromagnetic energy include _____
   A. radio waves.
   B. television waves.
   C. visible light.
   D. All of the above

7. _____ is the process where atoms are changed into negatively or positively charged ions during radiation.
   A. Impulses
   B. Milliamperage
   C. Kilovoltage
   D. Ionization

8. Which of the following is not a characteristic of short, hard wavelengths? _____
   A. High frequency
   B. Low energy
   C. High penetrating power
   D. All of the above

9. _____ radiation is the central beam that comes from the x-ray tubehead.
   A. Leakage
   B. Primary
   C. Scatter
   D. Secondary

10. _____ radiation is formed when the primary x-ray strikes or comes in contact with matter (any substance).
    - A. Leakage
    - B. Primary
    - C. Scatter
    - D. Secondary

11. _____ radiation is deflected from its path as it strikes matter.
    - A. Leakage
    - B. Primary
    - C. Scatter
    - D. Secondary

12. _____ radiation is a form of radiation that escapes in all directions from the tube or tubehead.
    - A. Leakage
    - B. Primary
    - C. Scatter
    - D. Secondary

13. The _____ equals the amount of radiation that will ionize one cubic centimeter of air.
    - A. rad
    - B. roentgen
    - C. rem
    - D. GY

14. The dose to which body tissues are exposed, measured in terms of its estimated biological effects, is called _____
    - A. Sv.
    - B. R.
    - C. GY.
    - D. mr.

15. The period of time between the exposure and development of biological effects is called the _____ period.
    - A. radiosensitive
    - B. sievert
    - C. latent
    - D. RBE

16. Name that portion of the dental x-ray unit where circuit boards and controls are located. _____
    - A. Milliamperage
    - B. Kilovoltage
    - C. Electronic timer
    - D. Control panel

17. The most common setting(s) for the kilovoltage is (are) _____
    - A. 30 kV.
    - B. 70 to 90 kV.
    - C. 10 to 15 kV.
    - D. 30 to 59 kV.

18. The most common settings for the milliamperage are _____
    - A. 10 to 15 mA.
    - B. 30 to 50 mA.
    - C. 70 to 90 mA.
    - D. 20 to 40 mA.

19. When current passes through the cathode filament and heats it to an extremely high temperature, this process is called _____
    - A. bisecting technique.
    - B. thermionic emission.
    - C. blurred image.
    - D. cross-section technique.

20. Which intraoral technique for film exposures does the American Association of Dental Schools and the American Academy of Oral and Maxillofacial Radiology recommend? _____
    - A. Paralleling
    - B. Bisecting
    - C. Horizontal
    - D. Occlusal

21. The _____ radiograph pictures the entire tooth and surrounding area.
    - A. bitewing
    - B. occlusal
    - C. periapical
    - D. edentulous

22. The _____ radiograph pictures the crowns, the interproximal spaces, and the crest area of the alveolar bone of both the maxillary and the mandibular teeth.
    - A. bitewing
    - B. occlusal
    - C. periapical
    - D. edentulous

23. The _____ radiograph pictures large areas of the mandible or maxilla (adult film size is #4).
    - A. bitewing
    - B. occlusal
    - C. periapical
    - D. edentulous

24. A clear film would indicate _____
    - A. double exposure.
    - B. no exposure.
    - C. underexposure.
    - D. overexposure.

25. When a film has been exposed to a high temperature followed by a low temperature, this is called _____
    - A. double exposure.
    - B. radiopaque.
    - C. fogged.
    - D. reticulation.

26. If the image on the film is light and a tire track pattern can be seen, the operator error was due to _____
    - A. the film being backward in the mouth.
    - B. double exposures.
    - C. underexposed film.
    - D. overexposed film.

27. _____ radiographs are used primarily by orthodontists to assess the patient's skeletal structure and profile.
    A. Bitewing   C. Occlusal
    B. Periapical   D. Cephalometric

28. _____ is used to locate and define lesions associated with the oral cavity.
    A. Digital imaging
    B. Magnetic resonance imaging
    C. Computed tomography
    D. Cephalometry

29. _____ is primarily used in diagnosis of temporomandibular joint disease.
    A. Digital imaging
    B. Magnetic resonance imaging
    C. Computed tomography
    D. Cephalometry

30. Electromagnetic radiation with short wavelengths with high frequency equals _____ energy.
    A. less   B. more

31. The D-speed film is called _____
    A. ektraspeed.   B. ultraspeed.

32. With the _____ technique for exposing occlusal radiographs, the central ray is directed perpendicular to the bisecting plane.
    A. cross-section   B. topographic

33. Which vertical angulation error is caused by not having enough angulation? _____
    A. Elongation   B. Foreshortening

34. When the cone is angled toward the mesial or the distal surfaces instead of the interproximal area, _____ occurs.
    A. cone cutting   B. overlapping

35. Which processing method reduces the processing time, with most processors being compact and some having daylight loading units? _____
    A. Automatic   B. Manual

36. Which processing solution chemically reduces the exposed area of the emulsion, making it visible to the naked eye? _____
    A. Developer   B. Fixer

37. Which processing solution removes the unexposed and undeveloped crystals from the film emulsion? _____.
    A. Developer   B. Fixer

38. The density of a structure determines to what degree x-rays penetrate it. Shades of dark gray to black would be interpreted as _____
    A. radiopaque.   B. radiolucent.

Radiation is divided into types. Match the type with its definition.

Type
39. _____ Primary
40. _____ Secondary
41. _____ Scatter
42. _____ Leakage

Definition
A. Escapes in all directions
B. Formed when primary x-ray strikes patient or comes in contact with matter
C. Central beam that comes from x-ray tubehead
D. Deflected from its path as it strikes matter

The x-ray tube is a vacuum tube. Match the components and their function.

Component
43. _____ Cathode
44. _____ Anode
45. _____ Filter
46. _____ Central beam
47. _____ Collimator

Function
A. Directs the flow of x-ray, made of tungsten target
B. Solid metal, made of aluminum
C. Lead diaphragm
D. Negative side where electrons will originate
E. Hard x-rays with short wavelengths

Dental intraoral film packets range in size according to specific radiographic exposures. Match the film size for its specific use.

Film Size

48. _____ No. 0
49. _____ No. 1
50. _____ No. 2
51. _____ No. 3
52. _____ No. 4

Use

A. Long bitewing film
B. Adult
C. Occlusal film
D. Narrow anterior film
E. Child

The direction of the central ray creates vertical angulation. The angulation will work with most patients. Match the area with vertical angulation.

Area

53. _____ Incisor/lateral
54. _____ Cuspids
55. _____ Bicuspids (premolars)
56. _____ Molars

Angulation

A. Maxillary +45°, Mandibular –20°
B. Maxillary +20°, Mandibular –5°
C. Maxillary +40°, Mandibular –15°
D. Maxillary +30°, Mandibular –10°

57. Some cells are more radiosensitive than others. Identify the most sensitive tissues and organs.
   1. Salivary glands
   2. Lymphoid
   3. Kidney
   4. Reproductive cells
   5. Intestinal epithelium
   6. Muscle
   7. Bone marrow
   8. Nerves

   A. 1, 3, 6, 8
   B. 1, 2, 3, 5
   C. 2, 4, 6, 8
   D. 2, 4, 5, 7

SKILL COMPETENCY ASSESSMENT

17-1 Radiography Infection Control

Student's Name _____ Date _____

Instructor's Name _____

SKILL Routine steps should be followed for all treatment areas to maintain absolute clinical asepsis. The patient is informed about the procedure.

PERFORMANCE OBJECTIVE The student will follow a routine procedure that meets the regulations and the protocol set forth by the dentist and regulatory agencies, keeping in mind that assistants' duties vary from state to state. The dental assistant checks with the dentist for instructions on which type of radiographs are needed for diagnosis. The assistant prepares the patient and area, takes the radiographs, and processes and mounts the films for viewing according to the infection control protocol.

	Self Evaluation	Student Evaluation	Possible Points	Instructor Evaluation	Comments
Equipment and Supplies					
1. Barriers for the x-ray room			2		
2. X-ray film (size selected accordingly)			2		
3. Rinn XCP materials (assembled for use) or other paralleling technique aids			2		
4. Film barriers (optional)			1		
5. Lead apron with thyroid collar			3		
6. Container for exposed film			2		
Competency Steps					
1. Wash and dry hands.			2		
2. Place appropriate barriers on dental chair, film, and x-ray equipment.			2		
3. Prepare equipment and supplies needed for procedure: sterile Rinn XCP instruments, tissue or a paper towel, cup or container with patient's name.			3		
4. After patient is seated and positioned (lead apron), place on glasses and mask and wash and dry hands. Don treatment gloves.			3		
5. After x-rays are exposed and removed from patient's mouth, wipe them off and place in a cup/container or on a covered surface.			3		
6. When all x-ray exposures are complete, remove lead apron from patient, following aseptic protocol (methods include removing with contaminated gloves on and disinfecting apron or removing contaminated gloves or placing on overgloves and removing apron).			2		
7. After patient is dismissed, remove and dispose of all barriers.			2		

17-1 continued

	Self Evaluation	Student Evaluation	Possible Points	Instructor Evaluation	Comments
8. Any areas that were not covered with a barrier must be disinfected, including x-ray film.			3		

TOTAL POINTS POSSIBLE	32	
TOTAL POINTS POSSIBLE—2nd Attempt	30	
TOTAL POINTS EARNED	_____	

Points assigned reflect importance of step to meeting objective: Important = 1; Essential = 2; Critical = 3. Students will lose 2 points for repeated attempts. Failure results if any of the critical steps are omitted or performed incorrectly. If using a 100-point scale, determine score by dividing points earned by total points possible and multiplying the results by 100.

SCORE: _____

SKILL COMPETENCY ASSESSMENT

17-2 Full-Mouth X-Ray Exposure with Paralleling Technique

Student's Name _____ Date _____

Instructor's Name _____

SKILL   Routine steps should be followed for all treatment areas to maintain absolute clinical asepsis. The patient is informed about the procedure. This procedure will include film placement and exposure for the central incisors in each arch and one-half of the maxillary arch and one-half of the mandibular arch. The same technique would be used to expose the opposite arches.

PERFORMANCE OBJECTIVE   The dental assistant will follow a routine procedure that meets the regulations and the protocol set forth by the dentist and regulatory agencies, keeping in mind that assistants' duties vary from state to state. The dental assistant checks with the dentist for the request that a full mouth set of radiographs be taken. The dental assistant prepares the equipment (Rinn XCP instruments), area, and the patient; takes the radiographs; and processes and mounts the films for viewing according to the infection control protocol.

	Self Evaluation	Student Evaluation	Possible Points	Instructor Evaluation	Comments
Equipment and Supplies					
1. Barriers for the x-ray room and equipment			2		
2. X-ray film (appropriate size and number of films)			2		
3. X-ray film barriers (optional)			1		
4. Cotton rolls (optional)			1		
5. Rinn XCP materials (assembled for use) or other paralleling technique aids			2		
6. Lead apron with thyroid collar			3		
7. Container for exposed film			2		
8. Paper towel or tissue			1		
Competency Steps					
1. Review patient's chart.			3		
2. Wash and dry hands.			2		
3. Place appropriate barriers on dental chair, film, and x-ray equipment.			2		
4. Prepare equipment and supplies needed for procedure, including sterile Rinn XCP instruments, tissue or paper towel, cup or container with patient's name.			3		
5. Turn x-ray machine on and check the mA, kV, and exposure time.			3		
6. Seat and position patient in an upright position.			2		
7. Have patient remove any removable appliances, earrings, or eyeglasses that may interfere with the exposing process.			2		
8. Place lead apron with the thyroid collar on patient.			3		

17-2 continued

	Self Evaluation	Student Evaluation	Possible Points	Instructor Evaluation	Comments
9. After patient is prepared, wash and dry hands and don latex treatment gloves.			3		

TOTAL POINTS POSSIBLE	37
TOTAL POINTS POSSIBLE—2nd Attempt	35
TOTAL POINTS EARNED	_____

Points assigned reflect importance of step to meeting objective: Important = 1; Essential = 2; Critical = 3. Students will lose 2 points for repeated attempts. Failure results if any of the critical steps are omitted or performed incorrectly. If using a 100-point scale, determine score by dividing points earned by total points possible and multiplying the results by 100.

SCORE: _____

SKILL COMPETENCY ASSESSMENT

17-3 Exposing Occlusal Radiographs

Student's Name _____ Date _____

Instructor's Name _____

SKILL Routine steps should be followed for all treatment areas to maintain absolute clinical asepsis. The patient is informed about the procedure. This procedure will include technique selection determined by the view the dentist needs for diagnosis (topographic or cross-section).

PERFORMANCE OBJECTIVE The dental assistant will follow a routine procedure that meets the regulations and the protocol set forth by the dentist and regulatory agencies, keeping in mind that assistants' duties vary from state to state. The dental assistant checks with the dentist for the request of technique selection to be taken. The dental assistant prepares the equipment and supplies, area, and the patient; takes the radiographs; and processes and mounts the films for viewing according to the infection control protocol.

	Self Evaluation	Student Evaluation	Possible Points	Instructor Evaluation	Comments
Equipment and Supplies					
1. Barriers for the x-ray room			2		
2. Occlusal film (#2 for children and #4 for adults)			2		
3. Lead apron with thyroid collar			3		
4. Container or barrier for exposed film			2		
Competency Steps					
1. Wash and dry hands.			2		
2. Place appropriate barriers.			2		
3. Prepare film, tissue or paper towel, and cup or container with patient's identification on it.			2		
4. Seat the patient in an upright position and place lead apron on patient.			3		
5. Wash and dry hands and don treatment gloves.			2		
Topographic Technique					
6. **For maxillary view**, patient is positioned so maxillary arch is parallel to the floor. Positioning is similar to that used for the bisecting technique.			3		
7. Film is placed in mouth with smooth/plain side toward the cone.			3		
8. Have patient close on the film, leaving about 2 mm of an edge beyond the incisors.			2		
9. Move cone to a vertical angulation of +65° to +75°.			2		
10. Direct cone over the bridge of nose, with lower edge of cone covering the incisors.			2		
11. **For mandibular view** using the topographic technique, patient's head is tilted back.			2		

17-3 continued

	Self Evaluation	Student Evaluation	Possible Points	Instructor Evaluation	Comments
12. Place smooth side of film on occlusal surfaces of teeth with central incisors at front edge of film.			2		
13. Have patient close gently on film.			1		
14. Vertical angulation will vary with each patient between −45° degree and −55°.			1		
15. Center cone over the film, directing central ray at middle and tip of the chin.			2		
Cross-Section Technique					
1. **For maxillary view** using this technique, the patient should be in an upright position, head tilted slightly back.			2		
2. Film placement is the same as that of topographic technique. Cone is positioned over the top of patient's head with central ray directed perpendicular to film.			2		
3. Be sure cone covers the maxillary area to be exposed.			2		
4. **For mandibular view**, the patient's head should be tilted back.			2		
5. Film placement is the same as with the topographic technique.			2		
6. Cone is positioned under the patient's chin with central ray directed perpendicular to the film. Patient may have to lift the chin up in order to position the cone.			2		
TOTAL POINTS POSSIBLE			52		
TOTAL POINTS POSSIBLE—2nd Attempt			50		
TOTAL POINTS EARNED			_____		

Points assigned reflect importance of step to meeting objective: Important = 1; Essential = 2; Critical = 3. Students will lose 2 points for repeated attempts. Failure results if any of the critical steps are omitted or performed incorrectly. If using a 100-point scale, determine score by dividing points earned by total points possible and multiplying the results by 100.

SCORE: _____

SKILL COMPETENCY ASSESSMENT

17-4 Processing Radiographs Using a Manual Tank
(corresponds to textbook Procedure 17-5)

Student's Name _____ Date _____

Instructor's Name _____

SKILL   Routine steps should be followed for all treatment areas to maintain absolute clinical asepsis. The dental assistant prepares the equipment and supplies and the area. The dental assistant takes the exposed radiographs to the darkroom to process. The processing area is to be well ventilated and exclude all white light.

PERFORMANCE OBJECTIVE   The dental assistant will follow a routine procedure that meets the regulations and the protocol set forth by the dentist and regulatory agencies, keeping in mind that assistants' duties vary from state to state. The dental assistant will process (develop, fix, and wash) the dental x-rays according to infection control protocol.

	Self Evaluation	Student Evaluation	Possible Points	Instructor Evaluation	Comments
Equipment and Supplies					
1. Barriers for the darkroom counter			2		
2. Exposed radiographs			2		
3. X-ray rack			1		
4. Processing tank			1		
5. Safety light			1		
6. Timer			1		
7. Thermometer			1		
8. Pencil			1		
9. Electric film dryer			1		
Competency Steps					
1. Wash and dry hands (gloves must be worn if x-rays are contaminated).			2		
2. Place barriers on clean surface in darkroom.			2		
3. Check temperature of developer with thermometer (check processing chart for corresponding temperature and time).			2		
4. Check volume of processing solutions and replenish if necessary.			2		
5. Stir developer and fixer if first processing that morning or afternoon. Stir with corresponding rods to match solutions—don't mix.			3		
6. Check x-ray rack that clips are working.			2		
7. Label x-ray rack in pencil with patient's name, date of exposure, and number of x-rays taken.			3		
8. Turn on safelights and turn off white lights.			3		
9. Remove films from wrappers and place on x-ray racks. Maintain absolute asepsis.			2		

17-4 continued (corresponds to textbook Procedure 17-5)

	Self Evaluation	Student Evaluation	Possible Points	Instructor Evaluation	Comments
10. Check film to ensure it is attached securely and placed in parallel manner, not touching adjacent film.			2		
11. Place into developer tank, agitate the rack to eliminate bubbles on surface of emulsion.			2		
12. Place tank cover on processing tank. Set timer for four and one-half minutes if temperature is at 68° in the developer. Clean up area and dispose of barriers and wrappers.			2		
13. When timer goes off, remove the x-ray rack from developer, letting the excess solution drip into the developer prior to placing the rack into running water. Let it rinse for thirty seconds.			2		
14. Remove x-ray rack from the rinsing, let the excess water drip off, and then immerse the rack into the fixing solution for ten minutes (quick fix for dentist can be three minutes and then return film for the remaining time).			3		
15. Replace the processing lid and set the timer for ten minutes.			3		
16. When ten minutes has lapsed, remove the x-ray rack of films from the fixer and place into the running water. Final wash takes twenty minutes.			2		
17. After twenty minutes, the rack of x-rays can be removed from the water and placed into an x-ray dryer for an additional fifteen to twenty minutes or until drying is completed.			2		
18. When x-rays are dry, remove from rack and place in labeled x-ray mount.			2		

TOTAL POINTS POSSIBLE   52

TOTAL POINTS POSSIBLE—2nd Attempt   50

TOTAL POINTS EARNED   _____

Points assigned reflect importance of step to meeting objective: Important = 1; Essential = 2; Critical = 3. Students will lose 2 points for repeated attempts. Failure results if any of the critical steps are omitted or performed incorrectly. If using a 100-point scale, determine score by dividing points earned by total points possible and multiplying the results by 100.

SCORE: _____

SKILL COMPETENCY ASSESSMENT

17-5 Processing Radiographs Using an Automatic Processor
(corresponds to textbook Procedure 17-6)

Student's Name _____ Date _____

Instructor's Name _____

SKILL Routine steps should be followed for all treatment areas to maintain absolute clinical asepsis. The dental assistant prepares the equipment and supplies and the area. The dental assistant takes the exposed radiographs to the automatic processor to process.

PERFORMANCE OBJECTIVE The dental assistant will follow a routine procedure that meets the regulations and the protocol set forth by the dentist and regulatory agencies, keeping in mind that assistants' duties vary from state to state. The dental assistant will process (develop, fix, wash, and dry) the dental x-rays according to infection control protocol.

	Self Evaluation	Student Evaluation	Possible Points	Instructor Evaluation	Comments
Equipment and Supplies					
1. Exposed radiographs			2		
2. Automatic x-ray processor with day loader			2		
Competency Steps					
1. Turn on automatic x-ray processor at beginning of each day.			2		
2. Wash and dry hands.			2		
3. Place exposed radiographs in the daylight loader with two additional containers.			2		
4. Place on gloves and position gloved hands through sleeves of the loader.			2		
5. Remove each radiograph from its packet, place film into container not contaminated. Do not touch and contaminate film as packet is removed.			3		
6. Place empty packets in contaminated cup.			2		
7. After all x-rays are unwrapped, remove gloves and place them in contaminated container.			2		
8. With clean hands, feed the unwrapped films into machine *slowly*. Start on one side of the processor and rotate to the other side. Repeat. If using a film holder, place all films in holder and release for processing. Continue until all films are processed. Maintain absolute asepsis.			3		
9. Remove processed films from outlet area and place in a labeled x-ray mount.			2		

TOTAL POINTS POSSIBLE   24

TOTAL POINTS POSSIBLE—2nd Attempt   22

TOTAL POINTS EARNED   _____

Points assigned reflect importance of step to meeting objective: Important = 1; Essential = 2; Critical = 3. Students will lose 2 points for repeated attempts. Failure results if any of the critical steps are omitted or performed incorrectly. If using a 100-point scale, determine score by dividing points earned by total points possible and multiplying the results by 100.

SCORE: _____

SKILL COMPETENCY ASSESSMENT

| **17-6** Processing Duplicating Technique *(corresponds to textbook Procedure 17-7)*

Student's Name _____ Date _____

Instructor's Name _____

SKILL   The dental assistant prepares the equipment and supplies and the area. Copies of x-rays can be made by a duplication process in the darkroom.

PERFORMANCE OBJECTIVE   The dental assistant will follow a routine procedure that meets the regulations and the protocol set forth by the dentist and regulatory agencies, keeping in mind that assistants' duties vary from state to state. The radiographs to be duplicated are taken to the darkroom by the dental assistant to duplicate.

	Self Evaluation	Student Evaluation	Possible Points	Instructor Evaluation	Comments
Equipment and Supplies					
1. Radiographs			2		
2. X-ray duplicating machine			2		
3. Automatic x-ray processor with daylight loader			2		
Competency Steps					
1. Place x-rays in desired position on duplicator, dot upward.			3		
2. If machine has a viewing light, turn it on to assist in placement of x-rays.			2		
3. Under safelight conditions, place duplicating film over the x-rays with emulsion side facing downward, contacting the x-ray (notch will be in upper left corner).			3		
4. Cover lid and latch tightly. Set timer to four to five seconds (can vary with machines).			2		
5. Activate machine to expose film.			2		
6. When completed, remove duplicating film under safelight conditions and process film.			2		

TOTAL POINTS POSSIBLE   20

TOTAL POINTS POSSIBLE—2nd Attempt   18

TOTAL POINTS EARNED   _____

Points assigned reflect importance of step to meeting objective: Important = 1; Essential = 2; Critical = 3. Students will lose 2 points for repeated attempts. Failure results if any of the critical steps are omitted or performed incorrectly. If using a 100-point scale, determine score by dividing points earned by total points possible and multiplying the results by 100.

SCORE: _____

SKILL COMPETENCY ASSESSMENT

17-7 Mounting Radiographs (corresponds to textbook Procedure 17-8)

Student's Name _____ Date _____

Instructor's Name _____

SKILL   The dental assistant prepares the equipment and supplies and the area. It may take several practices, but soon the operator will be able to quickly identify any incorrectly mounted x-rays and place them correctly.

PERFORMANCE OBJECTIVE   This procedure is performed by the dental assistant. A viewbox may or may not be used when mounting the radiographs. The American Dental Association recommends that dental offices use the labial mounting.

	Self Evaluation	Student Evaluation	Possible Points	Instructor Evaluation	Comments
Equipment and Supplies					
1. Radiographs			3		
2. Lighted viewbox			2		
3. X-ray mount (full, 18 x-ray mount)			2		
4. Clean, dry surface			2		
Competency Steps					
1. Wash and dry hands, label x-ray mount with patient's name, date of exposure (in pencil).			3		
2. Turn on light x-ray viewbox (optional).			1		
3. Place radiographs on clean surface, all dots outward (convex) to view.			3		
4. Categorize all x-rays into three groups: bitewings (four in number), anteriors (six in number), and posterior (eight in number).			2		
5. Place bitewing x-rays in mount, dots convex, molars toward outside, bicuspids toward inside, x-rays mounted according to curve of the spee.			2		
6. Place anterior x-rays, with maxillary on upper, mandibular on lower. Incisal edges closest to each other in mount and roots positioned as they grow. Centrals placed in middle, cuspids on outer sides, maxillary centrals are much larger than mandibular.			2		
7. Place remaining posterior x-rays. Molars toward outside and bicuspids toward inside. Maxillary molars have three roots, mandibular have two roots. Biting surfaces more closely positioned.			2		
8. Review mounted x-rays to verify proper placement.			3		

TOTAL POINTS POSSIBLE   27

TOTAL POINTS POSSIBLE—2nd Attempt   25

TOTAL POINTS EARNED   _____

Points assigned reflect importance of step to meeting objective: Important = 1; Essential = 2; Critical = 3. Students will lose 2 points for repeated attempts. Failure results if any of the critical steps are omitted or performed incorrectly. If using a 100-point scale, determine score by dividing points earned by total points possible and multiplying the results by 100.

SCORE: _____

Endodontics

The student should strive to meet the following objectives and demonstrate an understanding of the facts and principles presented in this chapter:

1. Define endodontics and endodontist.
2. Describe pulpal and periapical disease.
3. Identify diagnostic procedures.
4. Identify instruments used in endodontic procedures and describe their functions.
5. Identify materials used in endodontics and describe their functions.
6. Describe endodontic procedures and the responsibilities of the dental assistant.
7. Explain surgical endodontic procedures and the instruments used.

SUMMARY

Endodontics is the branch of dentistry that deals with the diagnosis and treatment of diseases of the pulp and the periapical tissues. Procedures include diagnosis, root canal treatment, and periapical surgery.

The endodontist is assisted by the dental assistants who perform traditional assisting responsibilities in addition to expanded duties specific to endodontics as allowed by the state Dental Practice Act.

Endodontic diagnosis includes patient medical and dental history; clinical examination, including pulp testing; and review of communication if the patient is sent from a referring dentist.

KEY TERMS

abscess	hemisection	pulpotomy
apical periodontitis	intracanal instruments	radiographs
apicoectomy	irreversible pulpitis	reamers
barbed broaches	master cone	retrograde filling
cellulitis	non-vital pulp	reversible pulpitis
electric pulp tester	obturating	root amputation
endodontics	osteomyelitis	root canal sealer
exudate	percussion	rubber stops
files	periapical abscess	spreaders
fistula	pulpal necrosis	transillumination test
Glick #1	pulpectomy	vital pulp
gutta percha		

EXERCISES AND ACTIVITIES

1. Endodontics is the branch of dentistry that deals with and includes which of the following procedures? _____
   A. Diagnosis
   B. Root canal treatment
   C. Periapical surgery
   D. All of the above

2. An advanced stage of periapical infection that spreads into and throughout the bone is called _____
   A. periodontitis.
   B. osteomyelitis.
   C. cellulitis.
   D. pulpitis.

3. When the abscess spreads into the facial tissue, causing swelling and discomfort, this condition is called _____
   A. pulpitis.
   B. periodontal disease.
   C. cellulitis.
   D. apical periodontitis.

4. A localized destruction of tissue and accumulation of exudate in the periapical region is called a _____
   A. fistula type abscess.
   B. periapical abscess.
   C. pulpitis abscess.
   D. necrosis abscess.

5. Tapping on the occlusal or incisal surface of the tooth is what form of clinical testing? _____
   A. Transillumination
   B. Palpation
   C. Percussion
   D. Electrical

6. Tooth vitality can also be evaluated by the use of a strong fiberoptic light to transmit light through the crown of the tooth. This procedure is called _____
   A. an electrical pulp test.
   B. percussion.
   C. palpation.
   D. transillumination.

7. Intracanal instruments made of fine metal wire with tiny, sharp projections along the instrument shaft are called _____
   A. barbed broaches.
   B. files.
   C. reamers.
   D. Gates-Glidden drills.

8. What files are used only in a push and pull motion? _____
   A. K-type   C. Reamer
   B. Hedström   D. Broach

9. Which of the following are placed on reamers and files to mark the length of the root canal? _____
   A. Rubber stops
   B. File stops
   C. Endo stops
   D. Markers
   E. All of the above

10. The instrument used to remove excess gutta percha is called a _____
    A. spreader.   C. plugger.
    B. Glick #1.   D. spoon.

11. Which of the following instruments has a long, twisted shank and blades that are far apart and is used in a twisting motion? _____
    A. File   C. Reamer
    B. Broach   D. Gates-Glidden drill

12. A thermoplastic material that is flexible at room temperature and is used to fill the canal is called _____
    A. a rubber stop.
    B. a file stop.
    C. gutta percha.
    D. a marker.

13. This material, which comes in powder/liquid form, when mixed is thick in consistency, is used with obturating materials, and is inserted into the canal, is called _____
    A. gutta percha.
    B. sealer.
    C. paper points.
    D. marker.

14. What piece of equipment measures the distance to the apex of the tooth and displays the information on a digital readout? _____
    A. Vitality scanner
    B. Pulp tester
    C. Heating unit
    D. Apex finder

15. During what phase of endodontic treatment is the pulp canal restored by permanently being filled and sealed? _____
    A. Reversible pulpitis
    B. Pulpotomy
    C. Obturation
    D. Hemisection

16. The master cone material is called _____
    A. paper point.
    B. Lentulo spiral.
    C. calcium hydroxide.
    D. gutta percha.

17. In what procedure is the apex of the root and infection surrounding the area surgically removed? _____
    A. Amputation   C. Pulpectomy
    B. Hemisection   D. Apicoectomy

18. The retrograde filling materials that can be placed into the prepared cavity include _____
    A. amalgam.
    B. composite.
    C. gutta percha.
    D. All of the above.

19. Characteristics of intracanal instruments include which of the following? _____
    1. Precise diameters
    2. Precise lengths
    3. Made of stainless steel
    4. Made of nickel titanium alloy wire
    5. Gutta percha
    6. Flexible
    7. Fracture resistant
    8. Corrosion resistant

    A. 1, 2, 3, 4, 5, 6, 7, 8
    B. 1, 2, 3, 5, 8
    C. 1, 2, 3, 4, 6, 7, 8
    D. 1, 2, 5, 6, 7, 8

20. Which of the following steps are not a part of a general root canal therapy? _____
    1. Administer anesthetic.
    2. Laying a surgical flap.
    3. Isolate the area.
    4. Amputate the root.
    5. Gain access to the pulp.
    6. Locate canals.

    A. 1, 2, 3
    B. 2, 4
    C. 1, 3, 5
    D. 1, 3, 6

21. If the pulp is inflamed but able to heal when the irritant is removed, this is called _____
    A. irreversible pulpitis.
    B. reversible pulpitis.

22. If the inflammation continues until the pulpal tissue can not recover, this condition is called _____
    A. irreversible pulpitis.
    B. reversible pulpitis.

23. The death of the pulpal cells, often the result of irreversible pulpitis, is called _____
    A. apical periodontitis.
    B. pulpal necrosis.

24. _____ consists of numerous cells of the inflammatory process of chronic apical periodontitis. _____
    A. Granuloma   B. Osteomyelitis

25. The _____, a long, tapered, endodontic instrument that is pointed on the ends, is used to adapt the gutta percha into the canal.
    A. plugger   B. spreader

26. The _____, a long, tapered endodontic instrument that is flat on the ends, is used to condense the filling material.
    A. plugger   B. spreader

27. The endodontic handpiece is attached to a _____ handpiece.
    A. high-speed   B. low-speed

28. The removal of all pulpal tissues, beginning in the coronal portion of the tooth and terminating short of the apex in the root canal of the tooth, is called a _____
    A. pulpectomy.   B. pulpotomy.

29. The removal of the pulp in the coronal portion of the tooth, leaving the pulp in the root canal intact and vital, is called a _____
    A. pulpectomy.   B. pulpotomy.

30. The surgical removal of one root and the overlying crown is called a _____
    A. root amputation. B. hemisection.

31. The surgical procedure to remove one or more roots of a multirooted tooth, in which the root is removed at the point where the root meets the crown, is called _____
    A. root amputation. B. hemisection.

SKILL COMPETENCY ASSESSMENT

18-1 Electronic Pulp Testing

Student's Name _____ Date _____

Instructor's Name _____

SKILL   Routine steps should be followed for all treatment areas to maintain absolute clinical asepsis. The patient is informed about the procedure. The dental assistant performs traditional assisting responsibilities in addition to expanded duties specific to endodontics allowed by the state Dental Practice Act.

PERFORMANCE OBJECTIVE   The student will follow a routine procedure that meets the regulations and the protocol set forth by the dentist and regulatory agencies, keeping in mind that assistants' duties vary from state to state. The electronic pulp tester indicates whether the tooth is vital or non-vital. The current creates an electrical stimulus to the tooth and responses to the stimulus are compared to determine the pulp vitality.

	Self Evaluation	Student Evaluation	Possible Points	Instructor Evaluation	Comments
Equipment and Supplies					
1. Basic setup: mouth mirror, explorer, and cotton pliers			3		
2. Electronic pulp tester			3		
3. Conducting medium, such as toothpaste			2		
Competency Steps					
1. Place small amount of toothpaste on tip of electrode.			2		
2. Dry tooth before using electrode.			3		
3. Ask patient to signal when they notice a sensation, usually a tingling or hot feeling.			3		
4. Place tip on facial surface of tooth and gradually increase the power. **Caution:** do not place electrode on a metal restoration.			3		
5. If patient feels any sensation, some degree of tooth vitality is indicated. If no sensation is felt, the pulp may be necrotic.			3		

TOTAL POINTS POSSIBLE   22

TOTAL POINTS POSSIBLE—2nd Attempt   20

TOTAL POINTS EARNED   _____

Points assigned reflect importance of step to meeting objective: Important = 1; Essential = 2; Critical = 3. Students will lose 2 points for repeated attempts. Failure results if any of the critical steps are omitted or performed incorrectly. If using a 100-point scale, determine score by dividing points earned by total points possible and multiplying the results by 100.

SCORE: _____

SKILL COMPETENCY ASSESSMENT

18-2 Root Canal Treatment

Student's Name _____ Date _____

Instructor's Name _____

SKILL   Routine steps should be followed for all treatment areas to maintain absolute clinical asepsis. The patient is informed about the procedure. The dental assistant performs traditional assisting responsibilities in addition to expanded duties specific to endodontics allowed by the state Dental Practice Act.

PERFORMANCE OBJECTIVE   The student will follow a routine procedure that meets the regulations and the protocol set forth by the dentist and regulatory agencies, keeping in mind that assistants' duties vary from state to state. The following sequence will indicate steps involved in a root canal treatment that requires two appointments. (Each office has a routine procedure that is carefully followed to ensure all pertinent information is gathered for endodontic diagnosis and treatment.)

	Self Evaluation	Student Evaluation	Possible Points	Instructor Evaluation	Comments
Equipment and Supplies					
1. Basic setup: mouth mirror, explorer, and cotton pliers			3		
2. Endodontic explorer and spoon excavator			2		
3. Locking cotton pliers			2		
4. Saliva ejector, evacuator tip (HVE), air-water syringe tip			3		
5. Cotton rolls, cotton pellets, and gauze sponges			3		
6. Anesthetic setup			3		
7. Dental dam setup			3		
8. High-speed handpiece and assortment of burs			3		
9. Low-speed handpiece			2		
10. Irrigating syringe and solution (sodium hypochlorite or hydrogen peroxide)			3		
11. Barbed broach, assorted reamers and files, and rubber stops			3		
12. Paper points (assortment)			2		
13. Temporization materials			2		
14. Permanent obturating materials (gutta percha or silver points and root canal sealer)			2		
15. Heat source			2		
16. Endodontic spreaders, pluggers, and the Glick #1			3		
17. Articulating forceps and paper			2		
Competency Steps					
Administer Anesthetic					
1. Administer topical and local anesthetic.			2		

18-2 continued

	Self Evaluation	Student Evaluation	Possible Points	Instructor Evaluation	Comments
2. After first appointment anesthetic may be unnecessary; the dentist will determine.			2		
3. Prepare the syringe and assist during administration of anesthetic.			3		
Isolate the Area					
1. Preparation for isolation of tooth for treatment.			3		
2. Place dental dam on selected tooth being endodontically treated.			3		
3. After dental dam placement, area should be wiped with disinfectant.			2		
Gain Access to the Pulp					
1. Dentist uses high-speed handpiece and bur to gain access to pulp. Opening is through crown and to expose the pulp chamber.			2		
2. Evacuate and maintain good visibility for the dentist.			2		
3. Once access to pulp, endodontic explorer is used to locate main and accessory canals.			2		
Remove the Pulpal Tissues					
1. Dentist will insert barbed broach into canal and withdraw pulpal tissue.			2		
2. Receive the barbed broach in a gauze sponge.			2		
Enlarge and Smooth the Root Canal					
1. Using x-ray, dentist estimates length of root of tooth. An apex finder may also be used. Rubber stops used to mark length of tooth on files/reamers. Series of small files to remove debris and enlarge canals (must be at least #25 file before Gates-Glidden burs can be used). As files enlarge the diameter of canal, the size of files and/or Gates burs increases.			3		
2. Prepare the stops on files and reamers. The dentist instructs the dental assistant to place rubber stops according to the measurement and precisely for each hand instrument. Keep the files and reamers in order and free from debris (duties vary depending on preferences of dentists; some dentists may want the assistant to sterilize reamers and files chairside, or they may request radiographs taken periodically).			3		
Irrigate the Root Canal					
1. Periodically, canal is irrigated to remove debris. After canal is flushed, it is dried with paper points.			2		
2. Prepare the irrigating solution in the disposable syringe and transfer to the operator. Operator					

18-2 continued

	Self Evaluation	Student Evaluation	Possible Points	Instructor Evaluation	Comments
flushes the solution into canal, the assistant evacuates the area. Then, transfer paper points in locking pliers to operator and receive the used saturated points in a gauze sponge.			2		
3. **Note:** The dentist may decide to place a temporary restoration and reappoint patient in several days. Prepare the temporary restorative materials and either place the temporary or assist the dentist in placement. Remove the dental dam and dismiss the patient.			2		

Obturate the Root Canal

	Self Evaluation	Student Evaluation	Possible Points	Instructor Evaluation	Comments
1. Obturation of the root canal is routinely performed at second appointment. After seating the patient, temporary is removed and canal is flushed.			2		
2. Radiographs are taken periodically throughout procedure for dentist to evaluate progress. Once canal is adequately enlarged and free of disease, it is permanently filled.			2		
3. Materials and techniques available to fill canal may vary, but gutta percha materials are most common.			2		
4. The dentist selects gutta percha point as the **master cone**. Cone no more than 1 mm short of prepared length. The dentist inserts cone in canal to check fit. If master cone is correct length and fits snugly near the apex, the cone is removed and the root canal sealer is prepared.			2		
5. Root canal sealer is mixed and placed in canal with a Lentulo spiral. The master cone is dipped into sealer and placed in canal.			2		
6. A spreader is used to create space for additional accessory gutta percha cone. Dip each accessory gutta percha cone into the root canal sealer and pass it to the dentist for placement. The spreader is passed to create space for subsequent cones. This procedure is repeated until canal is filled.			2		
7. Once canal is filled, excess gutta percha in the crown of the tooth is removed with a hot Glick #1 or a heated plugger. The warm gutta percha is vertically condensed into the cervical portion.			2		
8. Hold a 2 x 2 gauze to remove any excess gutta percha from the instruments.			2		
9. The final radiograph is taken.			3		
10. The coronal portion of the tooth is sealed with a permanent restoration or temporary restoration if a fixed prosthesis is the treatment of choice.			2		
11. The dental dam is removed and patient mouth is rinsed.			2		

18-2 continued

	Self Evaluation	Student Evaluation	Possible Points	Instructor Evaluation	Comments
12. The patient's occlusion is checked with articulating paper.			2		
13. Give the patient postoperative instructions and dismiss him or her.			2		

TOTAL POINTS POSSIBLE   107

TOTAL POINTS POSSIBLE—2nd Attempt   105

TOTAL POINTS EARNED   _____

Points assigned reflect importance of step to meeting objective: Important = 1; Essential = 2; Critical = 3. Students will lose 2 points for repeated attempts. Failure results if any of the critical steps are omitted or performed incorrectly. If using a 100-point scale, determine score by dividing points earned by total points possible and multiplying the results by 100.

SCORE: _____

Oral and Maxillofacial Surgery

OBJECTIVES

The student should strive to meet the following objectives and demonstrate an understanding of the facts and principles presented in this chapter:

1. Describe the scope of oral and maxillofacial surgery.
2. Identify the various surgical instruments used in this type of surgery and describe their functions.
3. Explain aseptic procedures followed in the oral surgeon's office.
4. Describe the evaluation procedures for new patients.
5. Describe how to prepare the patient for surgical treatment.
6. Explain surgical procedures, including tray setups and assisting responsibilities.
7. List postoperative instructions given to patients.
8. List and describe the types of dental implants and explain the procedures they are used with.
9. Explain the oral surgeon's relationship with the hospital.

SUMMARY

The dental surgery team may vary according to the goals of the surgeon concerning the practice. In addition to the oral and maxillofacial surgeon, the team usually consists of the receptionist, the business office staff, the dental assistants, and, in some offices, a nurse or an anesthesiologist.

The surgical dental assistant's responsibilities often vary depending on the size of the practice. The option to become a Certified Dental Assistant in Oral and Maxillofacial Surgery (COMSA) is available upon successful completion of an examination administered by the Dental Assisting National Board.

KEY TERMS

alveolitis	informed consent	root tip picks
alveoplasty	luxates	subperiosteal implant
biopsy	maxillofacial	surgical aspirating tips
dental implants	mouth props	surgical bone files
elevators	mucoperiosteum	surgical chisels
endosteal implants	needle holders	surgical curettes
excisional biopsy	orthognathic surgery	surgical mallet
exfoliative cytology	osseointegration	surgical scalpels
extraction forceps	periosteal elevator	surgical scissors
hemostats	retractors	tissue forceps
incisional biopsy	rongeurs	

EXERCISES AND ACTIVITIES

1. Oral and maxillofacial surgery involves surgery for _____
   A. functional malformations.
   B. facial injuries.
   C. facial esthetics.
   D. All of the above

2. The surgical dental assistant would perform the following skills as described in this text except _____
   A. transferring instruments.
   B. administering local anesthetic.
   C. maintaining the operating field during procedures.
   D. taking vital signs.

3. Which of the following instruments has straight, short beaks and fine serrations with a groove down the center of each beak and comes in a variety of sizes? _____
   A. Hemostat
   B. Needle holder
   C. Surgical scissors
   D. Rongeurs

4. Which of the following instruments has long serrated or grooved beaks and working ends that can be straight or curved and is used to retract tissue or grasp loose objects? _____
   A. Surgical scissors
   B. Needle holder
   C. Hemostat
   D. Rongeur

5. Which of the following instruments has pointed beaks with either straight or angled blades and can cut sutures or trim soft tissue? _____
   A. Scalpel
   B. Hemostat
   C. Needle holder
   D. Surgical scissors

6. Which of the following instruments is available in either beveled or bi-beveled sides, can be used alone if bone is soft, and removes or shapes the bone? _____
   A. Mallet   C. Rongeur
   B. File   D. Chisel

7. Which of the following instruments is usually double ended, comes in a variety of sizes and shapes, and is used in a back and forth motion to smooth the edges of alveolar bone? _____
   A. Mallet   C. Rongeur
   B. File   D. Chisel

8. When multiple teeth are removed, what instrument would be used to contour the remaining ridge of the alveolar bone and eliminate sharp edges? _____
   A. Surgical scissors
   B. File
   C. Rongeur
   D. Chisel

9. What hinged instrument is used to remove teeth from the alveolar bone? _____
   A. Apical elevator
   B. Periosteal elevator
   C. Extraction forceps
   D. Root tip pick

10. _____ is a contouring process in which sharp edges and points on the alveolar ridge are contoured and smoothed.
    A. Alveolitis   C. Exodontia
    B. Osseointegration   D. Alveoplasty

11. A non-surgical procedure that involves the oral surgeon removing a layer of cells from the surface lesion and spreading the gathered cells on a glass slab is called a(n) _____
    A. incisional biopsy.
    B. excisional biopsy.
    C. dental implant.
    D. exfoliative cytology.

12. The most common complication following an extraction is _____
    A. luxation.   C. alveolitis.
    B. alveoplasty.   D. exfoliative cytology.

13. The process in which a dental implant becomes fused with the bone and tissue is called _____
    A. orthognathic.   C. osseointegration.
    B. alveoplasty.   D. a stint.

14. The two most common dental implants are the subperiosteal and the endosteal. Which of the following are characteristics of a subperiosteal implant? _____
    1. Placed into the bone
    2. Often placed for denture patients
    3. Replaces a single tooth
    4. Most common on the mandibular
    5. Abutment posts are above the mucoperiosteum
    6. Require at least 2 mm ridge width
    7. Alveolar bone has atrophied
    8. Requires one or two surgeries

    A. 1, 2, 3, 4, 5, 6
    B. 1, 2, 5, 6
    C. 2, 3, 5, 8
    D. 2, 4, 7, 8

Following is a list of types of elevators. Match the elevator with its use.

Elevator
15. _____ Periosteal
16. _____ Elevator
17. _____ Apical
18. _____ Root tip picks

Use
A. Narrower blades, loosen root or bone fragments
B. Tease root tips or fragments, paired left/right
C. Detaches the periosteum or lifts mucoperiosteum
D. Single ended, T-shape handle, useful for variety of tasks

19. Surgical scalpels are used to incise the soft tissue and are then disposed of in the _____
    A. regular waste.   B. sharps container.

20. A retraction device used to grasp the tissue securely is called a _____
    A. cheek and lip retractor.
    B. tissue retractor.

21. A retractor that is spoon shaped or has a long blade and is placed between the border of the tongue and the lingual surfaces of the teeth is called a _____
    A. cheek and lip retractor.
    B. tongue retractor.

22. The _____ is composed of mucosa and periosteum.
    A. periosteum   B. mucoperiosteum

23. The term "luxates" would indicate what type of motion? _____
    A. Moves or dislocates
    B. Rocks back and forth

24. The term "subluxates" would indicate what type of motion? _____
    A. Moves or dislocates
    B. Rocks back and forth

25. When the oral surgeon removes a small section of the lesion and includes a small border of normal tissue, this is called an _____
    A. excisional biopsy. B. incisional biopsy.

SKILL COMPETENCY ASSESSMENT

19-1 Surgical Scrub

Student's Name _____ Date _____

Instructor's Name _____

SKILL Routine steps should be followed for all treatment areas to maintain absolute clinical asepsis. This procedure is performed by the dentist and the dental assistant before donning sterile gloves for a surgical procedure.

PERFORMANCE OBJECTIVE The student will follow a routine procedure that meets the regulations and the protocol set forth by the dentist and regulatory agencies, keeping in mind that assistants' duties vary from state to state. However, for oral surgery, the surgical hand scrub is completed before donning sterile gloves.

	Self Evaluation	Student Evaluation	Possible Points	Instructor Evaluation	Comments
Equipment and Supplies					
1. Antimicrobial soap			2		
2. Sterile scrub brush or foam sponge			2		
3. Disposable sterile towels			2		
Competency Steps					
1. Remove watch and rings before the scrub.			2		
2. Use an antimicrobial soap such as chlorhexidine gluconate.			2		
3. Wet hands and forearms up to the elbows with warm water.			3		
4. Dispense about 5 ml of soap into cupped hands and work into a lather.			2		
5. Beginning with the fingernails, scrub the fingers, hands, and forearms with surgical scrub brush.			3		
6. Rinse thoroughly with warm water.			2		
7. Repeat procedure with soap but without the scrub brush.			3		
8. Rinse with warm water, beginning at the fingertips and moving hands and forearms through the water and up so that the water drains off the forearms last.			3		

TOTAL POINTS POSSIBLE   26

TOTAL POINTS POSSIBLE—2nd Attempt   24

TOTAL POINTS EARNED   _____

Points assigned reflect importance of step to meeting objective: Important = 1; Essential = 2; Critical = 3. Students will lose 2 points for repeated attempts. Failure results if any of the critical steps are omitted or performed incorrectly. If using a 100-point scale, determine score by dividing points earned by total points possible and multiplying the results by 100.

SCORE: _____

SKILL COMPETENCY ASSESSMENT

19-2 Multiple Extractions and Alveoplasty (corresponds to textbook Procedure 19-3)

Student's Name _____ Date _____

Instructor's Name _____

SKILL   Routine steps should be followed for all treatment areas to maintain absolute clinical asepsis. Responsibilities of the dental assistant include evacuation and instrument transfer.

PERFORMANCE OBJECTIVE   The student will follow a routine procedure that meets the regulations and the protocol set forth by the dentist and regulatory agencies, keeping in mind that assistants' duties vary from state to state. This sterile procedure involves the removal of several teeth and contouring of the bone. The dental assistant must be prepared and be thinking ahead of the dentist. The assistant may be evaluated by performance, statement, and/or combined responses and action.

	Self Evaluation	Student Evaluation	Possible Points	Instructor Evaluation	Comments
Equipment and Supplies					
1. Basic setup: mouth mirror, explorer, and cotton pliers			3		
2. Gauze sponges			2		
3. Surgical HVE tip			2		
4. Luer lok syringe and sterile saline solution			2		
5. Retractor for the tongue and cheeks			3		
6. Local anesthetic			3		
7. Nitrous oxide setup (optional)			3		
8. Scalpel and blades			2		
9. Hemostat and tissue retractors			2		
10. Periosteal elevator			3		
11. Straight elevator			3		
12. Extraction forceps			3		
13. Surgical curette			3		
14. Root tip picks			3		
15. Rongeurs			3		
16. Bone file			3		
17. Low-speed handpiece and surgical burs			3		
18. Suture setup			3		
Competency Steps					
Inspection					
1. Transfer mirror, explorer to dentist.			2		
Anesthetic					
1. Patient may request general anesthesia. Prepare materials necessary.			3		

19-2 continued *(corresponds to textbook Procedure 19-3)*

	Self Evaluation	Student Evaluation	Possible Points	Instructor Evaluation	Comments
2. Patient may be required to have intravenous sedation. Prepare materials necessary.			3		
3. Prepare the materials necessary for local anesthetic.			3		
4. Assist in the administration of the anesthetic.			3		
Procedure					
1. The teeth are removed by the same technique described for the routine extraction.			3		
2. Pass the scalpel (state purpose).			3		
3. Evacuate area as necessary. Maintain operating field.			3		
4. Receive the scalpel.			3		
5. Pass periosteal elevator. State purpose.			3		
6. Use tissue forceps. State purpose.			3		
7. Maintain operating field.			3		
8. Transfer rongeurs. State purpose.			3		
9. Transfer low-speed handpiece with surgical burs.			3		
10. Keep the rongeurs and burs free of debris.			3		
11. Intermittently use the HVE and irrigation syringe with sterile saline solution.			3		
12. Maintain the operating field.			3		
13. Continue transfer of instruments as directed (final contouring, plastic stint try-in).			3		
14. Continue to maintain the surgical site.			3		
15. Remove the blood and debris from the stint between placements.			3		
Suturing					
1. Prepare the suture materials.			3		
2. Pass suturing material.			3		
3. Hold the flaps/tissue while dentist sutures.			3		
4. Prepare gauze pack.			2		
5. Gauze pack passed to dentist.			2		
6. Ready immediate denture.			2		
7. Pass immediate denture to dentist.			3		
8. Patient is given recovery time.			2		
9. Postoperative instructions are given both orally and written.			3		

19-2 continued *(corresponds to textbook Procedure 19-3)*

	Self Evaluation	Student Evaluation	Possible Points	Instructor Evaluation	Comments
10. Patient is scheduled for a postoperative examination and suture removal.			3		

TOTAL POINTS POSSIBLE	134
TOTAL POINTS POSSIBLE—2nd Attempt	132
TOTAL POINTS EARNED	_____

Points assigned reflect importance of step to meeting objective: Important = 1; Essential = 2; Critical = 3. Students will lose 2 points for repeated attempts. Failure results if any of the critical steps are omitted or performed incorrectly. If using a 100-point scale, determine score by dividing points earned by total points possible and multiplying the results by 100.

SCORE: _____

SKILL COMPETENCY ASSESSMENT

19-3 Removal of Impacted Third Molars (corresponds to textbook Procedure 19-4)

Student's Name _____ Date _____

Instructor's Name _____

SKILL   Routine steps should be followed for all treatment areas to maintain absolute clinical asepsis. This is a sterile procedure. The dental assistant transfers instruments and maintains the operating site.

PERFORMANCE OBJECTIVE   The student will follow a routine procedure that meets the regulations and the protocol set forth by the dentist and regulatory agencies, keeping in mind that assistants' duties vary from state to state. The procedure, bony impaction, is performed by the dentist. Because the teeth are impacted, the dentist will first have to expose the teeth by incising the tissue and removing the bone. The dental assistant must be prepared and be thinking ahead of the dentist. The assistant may be evaluated by performance, statement, and/or combined responses and actions.

	Self Evaluation	Student Evaluation	Possible Points	Instructor Evaluation	Comments
Equipment and Supplies					
1. Basic setup: mouth mirror, explorer, and cotton pliers			3		
2. Gauze sponges			2		
3. Surgical HVE tip			3		
4. Irrigating syringe and sterile saline solution			3		
5. Retractor for the tongue and cheeks			3		
6. Local anesthetic setup			3		
7. Nitrous oxide setup (optional)			3		
8. Scalpel and blades			2		
9. Hemostat and tissue retractors			2		
10. Periosteal elevator			3		
11. Straight elevator			3		
12. Extraction forceps (if needed)			3		
13. Root tip picks			3		
14. Surgical curette			3		
15. Rongeurs			3		
16. Bone file			3		
17. Low-speed handpiece and surgical burs			3		
18. Suture setup			3		
Competency Steps					
Anesthetic					
1. Patient may request general anesthesia. Prepare materials necessary.			3		
2. Patient may be required to have intravenous sedation. Prepare materials necessary.			3		
3. Prepare the materials necessary for local anesthetic.			3		

19-3 continued *(corresponds to textbook Procedure 19-4)*

	Self Evaluation	Student Evaluation	Possible Points	Instructor Evaluation	Comments
4. Assist in the administration of the anesthetic.			3		
Procedure					
1. Pass the scalpel (state purpose).			3		
2. Maintain operating field with surgical HVE.			3		
3. Receive the scalpel.			3		
4. Pass periosteal elevator. State purpose. And evacuate.			3		
5. Use tissue forceps. State purpose.			3		
6. Receive the periosteal elevator. And pass the handpiece and bur or the chisel.			3		
7. Pass elevators and forceps as the operator needs them. State purpose.			3		
8. Keep the area clear with HVE and periodically pass surgeon new gauze.			3		
9. Tooth is removed and examined to ensure all of the tooth has been removed.			3		
10. Transfer instruments and remove debris from the working ends with gauze.			3		
11. Prepare irrigating syringe with sterile water.			3		
12. Evacuate the site thoroughly.			3		
Suturing					
1. Prepare the suture materials.			3		
2. Place the suture in needle holder.			3		
3. Pass suturing material.			3		
4. Retract cheeks while oral surgeon sutures.			3		
5. Prepare gauze pack (moist, folded, and ready) following suturing.			2		
6. Gauze pack passed to dentist.			2		
Postsurgery					
1. Stay with patient during recovery.			3		
2. Patient is escorted when ready to leave.			3		
3. Ensure patient has necessary prescription(s).			3		
4. Postoperative instructions are given both orally and written.			3		

TOTAL POINTS POSSIBLE   124

TOTAL POINTS POSSIBLE—2nd Attempt   122

TOTAL POINTS EARNED   _____

Points assigned reflect importance of step to meeting objective: Important = 1; Essential = 2; Critical = 3. Students will lose 2 points for repeated attempts. Failure results if any of the critical steps are omitted or performed incorrectly. If using a 100-point scale, determine score by dividing points earned by total points possible and multiplying the results by 100.

SCORE: _____

SKILL COMPETENCY ASSESSMENT

19-4 Treatment for Alveolitis *(corresponds to textbook Procedure 19-6)*

Student's Name _____ Date _____

Instructor's Name _____

SKILL   Routine steps should be followed for all treatment areas to maintain absolute clinical asepsis. This is a sterile procedure. The dental assistant readies all materials as well as the tray setup.

PERFORMANCE OBJECTIVE   The student will follow a routine procedure that meets the regulations and the protocol set forth by the dentist and regulatory agencies, keeping in mind that assistants' duties vary from state to state. The assistant may be evaluated by performance, statement, and/or combined responses and action.

	Self Evaluation	Student Evaluation	Possible Points	Instructor Evaluation	Comments
Equipment and Supplies					
1. Basic setup: mouth mirror, explorer, and cotton pliers			3		
2. Surgical HVE tip			3		
3. Local anesthetic setup (may be required)			3		
4. Surgical scissors			3		
5. Surgical curettes			3		
6. Irrigating syringe and warm sterile saline solution			3		
7. Iodoform gauze or sponge			3		
Competency Steps					
Anesthetic					
1. Prepare the materials if necessary for local anesthetic.			3		
2. Assist in the administration of the anesthetic.			3		
Procedure					
1. Pass the suture scissors.			3		
2. Pass the surgical curette (state purpose).			3		
3. Prepare irrigating syringe.			3		
4. Maintain site area by retraction and suction.			3		
5. Prepare medicated dressing (state preparation).			3		
6. Pass dressing for surgeon placement.			3		
7. Give postoperative instructions (this includes doctor's prescription for pain control).			3		

19-4 continued *(corresponds to textbook Procedure 19-6)*

	Self Evaluation	Student Evaluation	Possible Points	Instructor Evaluation	Comments
8. Arrange for patient to return in one to two days to repeat the above process.			3		

TOTAL POINTS POSSIBLE   51

TOTAL POINTS POSSIBLE—2nd Attempt   49

TOTAL POINTS EARNED   _____

Points assigned reflect importance of step to meeting objective: Important = 1; Essential = 2; Critical = 3. Students will lose 2 points for repeated attempts. Failure results if any of the critical steps are omitted or performed incorrectly. If using a 100-point scale, determine score by dividing points earned by total points possible and multiplying the results by 100.

SCORE: _____

Oral Pathology

OBJECTIVES

The student should strive to meet the following objectives and demonstrate an understanding of the facts and principles presented in this chapter:

1. Define oral pathology and identify the dental assistant's role in this specialty.
2. Characterize the process of inflammation.
3. Identify oral lesions according to their placement.
4. Identify the oral diseases and the lesions related to biological agents.
5. Describe the oral diseases and the lesions related to physical agents.
6. Identify the oral diseases and the lesions related to chemical agents.
7. Identify the oral conditions related to hormonal disturbances.
8. Identify the oral conditions related to developmental disturbances.
9. Distinguish the oral conditions related to nutritional disturbances.
10. Identify the conditions and the lesions of oral neoplasms.
11. Identify the oral lesions related to HIV and AIDS.
12. Describe the conditions related to miscellaneous disorders affecting the oral cavity.

SUMMARY

The dental assistant, who sits opposite the dentist, has a different view of the patient's oral cavity. Anything that appears to be atypical should be brought to the dentist's attention, without alarming the patient.

The dental assistant does not diagnose oral pathological diseases but identifies abnormal conditions in the mouth. Further, the dental assistant must know how to prevent disease transmission, how the identified pathological condition may interfere with planned treatment, and what effect it will have on the overall health of the patient.

KEY TERMS

abscess
actinomycosis
angular cheilitis
ankylosis
anodontia
aphthous ulcers
biopsy
blister
bulla
candida albicans
canker sores
cleft lip
cleft palate

cyst
dysplasic cells
ecchymosis
etiology
fissured tongue
Fordyce's spots
granuloma
hematoma
herpes labialis
herpes zoster
herpetic gingivostomatitis
herpetic whitlow
histamine

human immunodeficiency
  virus (HIV)
hyperkeratinized
hyperplasia
inflammation
innocuous
Kaposi's sarcoma
lesions
macule
neonatal teeth
neoplasm
nodule
opportunistic infections

orifices
palpate
papule
patch
petechiae
plaque
purpura
pustule
supernumerary teeth
thrush
ulcer
vesicles
Wickham's striae

EXERCISES AND ACTIVITIES

1. Which agents may bring on a disease condition that exhibits signs within the oral cavity? _____
   A. Biological
   B. Physical
   C. Chemical
   D. All of the above

2. Which disturbances will also show disease signs within the mouth? _____
   A. Hormonal
   B. Developmental
   C. Nutritional
   D. All of the above

3. _____ is capable of causing the production of an antibody.
   A. Thrush
   B. An antigen
   C. A vesicle
   D. A cyst

4. An all-encompassing term for an abnormal structure in the oral cavity is _____
   A. plaque.   C. antigen.
   B. histamine.   D. lesion.

5. A dentist may _____ (feel with fingers) a suspicious lesion.
   A. biopsy   C. stretch
   B. edema   D. palpate

6. _____ is the surgical removal of a small amount of the suspicious lesion tissue.
   A. Etiology   C. Orifice
   B. Biopsy   D. Ankylosis

7. What lesion is caused by bleeding from a ruptured blood vessel during an injection of oral anesthetic? _____
   A. Cyst   C. Hematoma
   B. Blister   D. Nodule

8. A(n) _____ is a concentrated area of pus formed as a result of infection by microorganisms.
   A. abscess   C. cyst
   B. inflammation   D. blister

9. Which of the following lesions is associated with chronic inflammation and appears as a neoplasm that is filled with granulation tissue? _____
   A. Ecchymosis   C. Nodule
   B. Granuloma   D. Purpura

10. What infection, caused by a bacterium, is attributed to painful swelling at first and later pus and yellow granules discharging from the area? _____
    A. Herpes simplex
    B. Actinomycosis
    C. Herpes labialis
    D. Aphthous ulcer

11. The virus responsible for herpes simplex is transmitted through physical contact and is seen normally in children around the age of six as _____
    A. actinomycosis.
    B. herpes labialis.
    C. herpes zoster.
    D. herpetic gingivostomatitis.

12. What herpetic virus can cause a crusting ulceration on the fingers, hands, or eyes that is extremely painful? _____
    A. Herpes labialis
    B. Herpes zoster
    C. Aphthous ulcer
    D. Herpetic whitlow

13. _____ appears as painful lesions that can last up to five weeks, and patients with HIV are predisposed to it.
    A. Aphthous ulcer
    B. A canker sore
    C. Herpes simplex
    D. Herpes labialis
    E. Herpes zoster

14. What disease, caused by bacteria, has three primary stages, with bone and cartilage being destroyed in the final stage? _____
    A. Hutchinson's   C. Syphilis
    B. Mulberry   D. Thrush

15. The fungal infection of candidiasis in children, which appears as a white, thick covering over the oral mucosa, is commonly called _____
    A. a blister.
    B. thrush.
    C. a fissured tongue.
    D. a patch.

16. An ill-fitting denture can cause small ulcers that, after continued irritation, become folds of excess tissue called _____
    A. hypoplasia.   C. thrush.
    B. hyperplasia.   D. granuloma.

17. The heat and the irritating effect of chemicals in tobacco can cause areas of tissue to first turn red. If the irritation continues, the epithelium tissue builds up a layer of keratin as a protective coating; this tissue area is described as _____
    A. nicotine stomatitis.
    B. hyperkeratinized.
    C. hypokeratinized.
    D. aspirin burn.

18. The openings of the salivary glands are called _____
    A. infections.
    B. orifices.
    C. apexes.
    D. granulomas.

19. A condition in which the tooth, cementum, or dentin fuses with alveolar bone is called _____
    A. ankylosis.
    B. anodontia.
    C. dentinogenesis.
    D. germination.

20. Which of the following conditions occurs when teeth are congenitally missing? It can affect primary or permanent teeth or both and is most often seen in permanent third molars. _____
    A. Amelogenesis imperfecta
    B. Ankylosis
    C. Anodontia
    D. Macrodontia

21. Numerous light-yellow lesions are sometimes found in the oral cavity, most often on the buccal mucosa. These round lesions, which are sebaceous oil glands near the surface of the epithelium, are called _____
    A. exostoses.
    B. angular cheilitis.
    C. Fordyce's spots.
    D. dysplasic cells.

22. What developmental disturbance appears as a wrinkled, deeply grooved surface on the tongue? It may be symmetrical or irregular in pattern. _____
    A. Fissured tongue
    B. Ankyloglossia
    C. Black hairy tongue
    D. Bifid tongue

23. What condition will form a lesion in the corner of the mouth and is a result of vitamin B complex deficiency? _____
    A. Herpes labialis
    B. Herpetic zoster
    C. Angular cheilitis
    D. *Candida albicans*

24. When a patient loses vertical dimensions of the face, saliva can pool in the corners of the mouth, and a fungal infection can occur called _____
    A. herpes labialis.
    B. herpes zoster.
    C. angular cheilitis.
    D. *candida albicans.*

25. With a depressed immune system, _____ infections such as herpes, hepatitis, tuberculosis, candidosis, and pneumonia can overcome the individual's system.
    A. innocuous
    B. opportunistic
    C. hormonal
    D. chemical

26. An unusual malignant vascular tumor present in a number of AIDS patients is called _____
    A. herpetic whitlow.
    B. Kaposi's sarcoma.
    C. *candida albicans.*
    D. dysplasic cells.

27. Which of the following lesions, according to its placement in the surface of the oral mucosa, is classified as above the surface? _____
    A. Cyst
    B. Ecchymosis
    C. Nodule
    D. Blister

28. A hematoma lesion is classified as _____
    A. above the surface of the oral mucosa.
    B. below the surface of the oral mucosa.
    C. even with the surface of the oral mucosa.
    D. flat with the surface of the oral mucosa.

29. Which of the following lesions is classified as below the surface of the oral mucosa? _____
    A. Bulla
    B. Pustule
    C. Abscess
    D. Granuloma

30. A macule lesion is classified as _____
    A. above the surface of the oral mucosa.
    B. below the surface of the oral mucosa.
    C. even with the surface of the oral mucosa.
    D. flat with the surface of the oral mucosa.

31. Which conditions are an essential part of the body's response to injury or disease? _____
    1. Biological agents
    2. Redness (erythema)
    3. Chemical agents
    4. Heat
    5. Swelling (edema)
    6. Hormonal agents
    7. Pain
    8. Physical agents

    A. 1, 4, 5, 8
    B. 2, 4, 5, 7
    C. 1, 2, 3, 6
    D. 2, 3, 4, 6

32. Which of the following lesions can be classified as flat or above the surface of the oral mucosa? _____
    1. Granuloma
    2. Petechiae
    3. Purpura
    4. Bulla
    5. Blister
    6. Neoplasm
    7. Plaque
    8. Nodule

    A. 2, 3, 5
    B. 2, 3, 4
    C. 1, 6, 8
    D. 6, 7, 8

33. Canker sores are associated with which of the following? _____
    1. Abscess
    2. Heredity
    3. Trauma
    4. Plaque
    5. Stress
    6. Food allergens
    7. Hormonal changes
    8. Hematoma

    A. 1, 2, 4, 5, 8
    B. 2, 3, 5, 6, 7
    C. 2, 3, 4, 7, 8
    D. 1, 2, 3, 6, 7

34. Oral cancer warning signs include which of the following? _____
    1. Blister that is fluid filled and leaks into the blood vessels
    2. Sore in the oral cavity that does not heal within one month
    3. Lumps and swelling in the oral cavity, on the lips, or on the neck
    4. Concentrated area of pus from infection
    5. Lingual frenum attached too near the tip of the tongue
    6. White lesions or rough lesions in the mouth or on the lips

    A. 1, 3, 5
    B. 2, 3, 6
    C. 3, 4, 5
    D. 1, 2, 3

35. A bulla is a large (greater than one-half inch in diameter), fluid-filled blister _____
    A. above the surface of the oral mucosa.
    B. flat with the surface of the oral mucosa.

36. A papule, whose surface may be pigmented in color and either smooth or warty in texture, is a lesion that is _____
    A. flat with the surface of the oral mucosa.
    B. above the surface of the oral mucosa.

37. Ecchymosis, a medical term for bruising of the tissue, is _____
    A. even or flat with the surface of the oral mucosa.
    B. above the surface of the oral mucosa.

38. What virus is responsible for cold sores (painful blisters around the mouth), commonly called fever blisters? _____
    A. Aphthous ulcer
    B. Herpes simplex

39. The construction of an opturator is for treating which of the following developmental disturbances? _____
    A. Cleft lip   B. Cleft palate

40. Teeth that are present at the time of birth or within the first month after birth are called _____
    A. microdontia.   B. neonatal teeth.

41. Referred to as extra teeth, these teeth are seen most frequently in the maxillary anterior or in the third molar area, both maxillary and mandibular. _____
    A. Supernumerary teeth
    B. Microdontia teeth

Orthodontics

OBJECTIVES

The student should strive to meet the following objectives and demonstrate an understanding of the facts and principles presented in this chapter:

1. Define orthodontics and describe the orthodontic setting.
2. Define the role of the dental assistant in an orthodontic setting.
3. Define and describe occlusion and malocclusion.
4. Identify the causes of malocclusion.
5. Describe preventive, interceptive, and corrective orthodontics.
6. Explain the process of tooth movement.
7. Describe the preorthodontic appointment for the diagnostic records.
8. Describe the consultation appointment and the roles of the patient and the orthodontist.
9. Differentiate between fixed and removable appliances.
10. Identify and give the function of the basic orthodontic instruments.
11. Describe the stages of orthodontic treatment.
12. Explain the procedure for removing the orthodontic appliances and how the teeth are retained in position after removal of the appliances.

SUMMARY

The orthodontic team consists of the orthodontist, reception and business office staff, office coordinator, the orthodontic assistants, and laboratory technicians. The orthodontic assistant has a variety of responsibilities, depending on the size of the practice and the number of auxiliaries. The functions also vary with each state's Dental Practice Act.

To become a credentialed orthodontic assistant, a specialty examination must be passed.

KEY TERMS

activator
Angle's classification
arch wires
brackets
buccal tubes
buccoversion
corrective orthodontics
distoversion

elastics
fixed appliances
headgear
interceptive
ligature wire
linguoversion
malocclusion
normal occlusion

orthodontic bands
overbite
removable appliances
resorption
separators
space maintainer
springs

EXERCISES AND ACTIVITIES

1. What specialty of dentistry deals with recognition, prevention, and treatment of malalignment and irregularities of the teeth, jaws, and face? _____
   A. Endodontics
   B. Radiology
   C. Oral pathology
   D. Orthodontics

2. The orthodontic teams consist of the _____
   A. dentist.
   B. receptionist and business staff.
   C. assistant.
   D. laboratory technician.
   E. All of the above

3. Which orthodontic team member may pour and trim diagnostic models and construct orthodontic appliances? _____
   A. Laboratory technician
   B. Orthodontic assistant
   C. Office coordinator
   D. Business office staff

4. Which of the following is an ideal occlusion relationship? _____
   A. Transversion of a single tooth
   B. Labial or buccal version—toward the lip
   C. Maxillary and mandibular teeth are in maximum contact and normally spaced
   D. Infraversion in the arch

5. The established system to classify malocclusion is called _____ classification.
   A. transversion
   B. Angle's
   C. Pasteur's
   D. interceptive

6. A common treatment that is considered preventive or interceptive is _____
   A. treatment of adults.
   B. treatment of children in last stage of mixed dentition.
   C. treatment of children entering full permanent dentition.
   D. extraction of teeth to prevent overcrowding.

7. Common treatments that fall under corrective orthodontics include which of the following? _____
   A. Braces
   B. Bands
   C. Retainers
   D. Arch wires
   E. All of the above

8. The process that allows teeth to be moved by eliminating tissue no longer needed by the body is called _____
   A. deposition.
   B. resorption.
   C. buccoversion.
   D. linguoversion.

9. An example of a fixed orthodontic appliance is _____
   A. a retainer.
   B. an activator.
   C. braces.
   D. headgear.

10. What fixed appliance is either welded to the bands or bonded directly to the teeth? _____
    A. Band
    B. Bracket
    C. Buccal tube
    D. Ligature wire

11. The function of the _____ is to apply force to either move the teeth or hold them in the desired positions.
    A. buccal tubes
    B. bracket
    C. arch wire
    D. springs

12. The _____ wraps around the bracket and is tightened by twisting.
    A. arch wire
    B. ligature wire
    C. spring
    D. separator

13. _____ are attached to hooks or buttons that are secured on the band or brackets.
    A. Springs
    B. Tooth positioners
    C. Elastic separators
    D. Elastics

14. After the premature loss of a primary tooth, what special fixed appliance is worn to maintain a space for the permanent tooth? _____
    A. Bracket
    B. Space maintainer
    C. Headgear
    D. Activator

15. What removable appliance, usually worn for a specific number of hours each day, is used to apply force to move teeth, to restrain or alter cranial-facial bone growth, and to reinforce stability of intraoral appliances? _____
    A. Space maintainer
    B. Headgear
    C. Activator
    D. Tooth positioner

16. Normal occlusion is a general term that includes which of the following? _____
    1. Mandibular teeth are in maximum contact with maxillary teeth.
    2. Teeth are slightly rotated and turned.
    3. Teeth are mesial to normal position.
    4. Anterior teeth overlap 2 mm maxillary to mandibular.

    A. 1, 2, 3, 4
    B. 2, 3
    C. 1, 4
    D. 2, 3

17. The etiology of malocclusion can fall into one of three categories: genetic, systemic, or local. Genetic factors may be responsible for which of the following? _____
    1. Systemic diseases
    2. Trauma
    3. Palatal clefts
    4. Supernumerary teeth
    5. Thumb sucking
    6. Nutritional disturbances

    A. 1, 2
    B. 3, 4
    C. 5, 6
    D. 3, 6

18. _____ means the tooth is in a distal to normal position.
    A. Linguoversion   B. Distoversion

19. _____ means the tooth is tipped toward the lip or cheek.
    A. Torsoversion   B. Labioversion

20. What cause of malocclusio[n] disease and nutritional dis[ ] normal schedule of dentit[ ] infancy and early childho[od]
    A. Local factors   B[ ]

21. The teeth are retained in position through the _____ process, which creates and deposits new cells.
    A. resorption   B. deposition

22. _____ are placed in the contact areas between the teeth, forcing the teeth to spread apart to accommodate the orthodontic bands.
    A. Separators   B. Plastic rings

23. A(n) _____ is an abnormal relationship of a tooth or a group of teeth in one arch to the opposing teeth in the other arch.
    A. underjet   B. cross-bite

24. When the vertical overlap of the maxillary teeth is greater than the incisal one-third of the mandibular anterior teeth, this is termed _____
    A. overjet.   B. overbite.

25. An abnormal horizontal distance between the labial surface of the mandibular anterior teeth and the labial surface of the maxillary anterior teeth is called _____
    A. overjet.   B. overbite.

COMPETENCY ASSESSMENT

21-1 Placement and Removal of Elastic Separators

Student's Name _____ Date _____

Instructor's Name _____

SKILL   Routine steps should be followed for all treatment areas to maintain absolute clinical asepsis. The dental assistant must be prepared and thinking ahead to anticipate the dentist's needs. The elastic separators are small circles that are stretched for placement. They fit around the contact area and when released apply a constant pressure until the teeth move apart. The dental assistant may be permitted, in some states, to place and remove these separators.

PERFORMANCE OBJECTIVE   The student will follow a routine procedure that meets the regulations and the protocol set forth by the dentist and regulatory agencies, keeping in mind that assistants' duties vary from state to state. The assistant may be evaluated by performance, statement, and/or combined responses and action. After the diagnosis, the first treatment appointment is to place separators to prepare the teeth for the orthodontic bands. At the dentist's directions, the expanded-function assistant places the separators. The patient is scheduled in several days to have the separators removed and the bands placed.

	Self Evaluation	Student Evaluation	Possible Points	Instructor Evaluation	Comments
Equipment and Supplies					
1. Basic setup: mouth mirror, explorer, and cotton pliers			3		
2. Separation pliers			3		
3. Separators (wire or elastic)			3		
4. Dental floss or tape (optional technique)			2		
5. Scaler			3		
Competency Steps					
Placement of Elastic Separators with Separating Pliers					
1. Examine patient's mouth using the mouth mirror.			3		
2. Place elastic separator over beaks of the separating pliers.			3		
3. Squeeze the pliers to secure the elastic on the pliers.			3		
4. Further squeeze the pliers to stretch elastic separator.			3		
5. Place elastic between two teeth in a back-and-forth motion (similar to flossing).			3		
6. Insert one side of elastic band below contact in interproximal space.			3		
7. Release tension on separating pliers.			3		
8. Remove pliers.			3		
9. Repeat process on all interproximal spaces around teeth to receive metal bands.			3		
Placement of Separators with Dental Floss					
1. Place two lengths of dental floss through an elastic separator.			3		

21-1 continued

	Self Evaluation	Student Evaluation	Possible Points	Instructor Evaluation	Comments
2. Fold over each floss length until ends meet.			3		
3. Pull each piece of floss by ends to stretch elastic.			3		
4. Using the back-and-forth motion, insert separator.			3		
5. Once separator is in place, release floss and pull free.			3		
Removal of Elastic Separators					
1. Using a scaler or explorer, insert one end into ring of elastic separator.			3		
2. Place finger over top of separator to prevent separator from snapping and injuring the patient.			3		
3. Pull gently on instrument toward the occlusal until elastic is free of the contact.			3		

TOTAL POINTS POSSIBLE   65

TOTAL POINTS POSSIBLE—2nd Attempt   63

TOTAL POINTS EARNED   _____

Points assigned reflect importance of step to meeting objective: Important = 1; Essential = 2; Critical = 3. Students will lose 2 points for repeated attempts. Failure results if any of the critical steps are omitted or performed incorrectly. If using a 100-point scale, determine score by dividing points earned by total points possible and multiplying the results by 100.

SCORE: _____

SKILL COMPETENCY ASSESSMENT

21-2 Cementation of Orthodontic Bands *(corresponds to textbook Procedure 21-4)*

Student's Name _____ Date _____

Instructor's Name _____

SKILL   Routine steps should be followed for all treatment areas to maintain absolute clinical asepsis. The dental assistant must be prepared and thinking ahead to anticipate the dentist's needs. The assistant mixes cement according to manufacturer's directions and loads the first band. The dental assistant must position the bands so that the orthodontist can pick up the bands in the order of sequence of placement. The orthodontist seats the band on the tooth.

PERFORMANCE OBJECTIVE   The student will follow a routine procedure that meets the regulations and the protocol set forth by the dentist and regulatory agencies, keeping in mind that assistants' duties vary from state to state. The assistant may be evaluated by performance, statement, and/or combined responses and action. The orthodontic bands are prepared specifically for the patient. The orthodontist places the bands on the teeth to accomplish the task needed to correct the patient's malocclusion. The dental assistant mixes the cement and prepares the band for seating.

	Self Evaluation	Student Evaluation	Possible Points	Instructor Evaluation	Comments
Equipment and Supplies					
1. Basic setup: mouth mirror, explorer, and cotton pliers			3		
2. Cotton rolls and gauze			3		
3. Saliva ejector and HVE			3		
4. Slow-speed handpiece with rubber cup and prophy paste			3		
5. Selected and prepared bands			3		
6. Band pusher			3		
7. Bite stick			3		
8. Scaler			3		
9. Cement of choice			3		
10. Paper pad or glass slab			3		
11. Cement spatula			3		
12. Plastic filling instrument (PFI)					
Competency Steps					
1. Remove separators.			3		
2. Teeth are given a rubber cup polish.			3		
3. Patient's mouth is rinsed thoroughly.			3		
4. Teeth are dried and cotton rolls placed for isolation in areas where bands will be placed.			3		
5. Mix cement.			3		
6. Load cement in first band.			3		
7. Passing of bands made as easy as possible.			3		
8. Position bands so orthodontist can pick up bands in order of sequence of placement.			3		

21-2 continued *(corresponds to textbook Procedure 21-4)*

	Self Evaluation	Student Evaluation	Possible Points	Instructor Evaluation	Comments
9. Pass band driver.			3		
10. Band procedure is repeated until all bands have been cemented or until cement becomes too thick and a new mix is required.			3		
11. When new mix is required, clean instruments with wet gauze or alcohol wipe and mix additional cement.			3		
12. Cement is allowed to dry (clean up as in Step 11).			3		
13. After cement is set, remove excess cement with a scaler.			3		
14. When all cement has been removed, protective pins or wax is removed from brackets.			3		
15. The patient's mouth is rinsed.			2		

TOTAL POINTS POSSIBLE   77

TOTAL POINTS POSSIBLE—2nd Attempt   75

TOTAL POINTS EARNED   _____

Points assigned reflect importance of step to meeting objective: Important = 1; Essential = 2; Critical = 3. Students will lose 2 points for repeated attempts. Failure results if any of the critical steps are omitted or performed incorrectly. If using a 100-point scale, determine score by dividing points earned by total points possible and multiplying the results by 100.

SCORE: _____

SKILL COMPETENCY ASSESSMENT

21-3 Direct Bonding of Brackets *(corresponds to textbook Procedure 21-5)*

Student's Name _____ Date _____

Instructor's Name _____

SKILL Routine steps should be followed for all treatment areas to maintain absolute clinical asepsis. The dental assistant must be prepared and thinking ahead to anticipate the dentist's needs. The placement of brackets directly to the anterior teeth is a popular choice of treatment because they are more esthetic and easier to maintain good oral hygiene. The brackets are bonded to the tooth surface with a similar material and technique used to restore anterior teeth. The bonding material is prepared according to manufacturer's directions. The dental assistant must position the brackets so that the orthodontist can pick up the bracket in the order of sequence of placement. The orthodontist seats the bracket on the tooth.

PERFORMANCE OBJECTIVE The student will follow a routine procedure that meets the regulations and the protocol set forth by the dentist and regulatory agencies, keeping in mind that assistants' duties vary from state to state. The assistant may be evaluated by performance, statement, and/or combined responses and action. The orthodontic brackets are prepared specifically for the patient. The orthodontist places the brackets on the teeth to accomplish the task needed to correct the patient's malocclusion. This procedure involves bonding the brackets to the teeth; the dental assistant prepares the bracket for seating.

	Self Evaluation	Student Evaluation	Possible Points	Instructor Evaluation	Comments
Equipment and Supplies					
1. Basic setup: mouth mirror, explorer, and cotton pliers			3		
2. Cotton rolls and gauze			3		
3. Saliva ejector and HVE			3		
4. Slow-speed handpiece with rubber cup and pumice			3		
5. Bracket kit			3		
6. Retractors for the cheeks and lips			3		
7. Bracket forceps			3		
8. Acid etchant			3		
9. Bonding agent			3		
10. Scaler			3		
Competency Steps					
1. Polish teeth that are to receive brackets with rubber cup and pumice.			3		
2. Patient's mouth is rinsed and dried.			3		
3. Cotton rolls are placed in areas where brackets are to be bonded.			3		
4. Retractors are positioned.			3		
5. Prepare etchant.			3		
6. Pass etchant to operator.			3		
7. Acid etchant is placed on enamel surface (follow manufacturer's directions for time).			3		
8. Maintain operating field so that it stays dry.			3		

21-3 continued *(corresponds to textbook Procedure 21-5)*

	Self Evaluation	Student Evaluation	Possible Points	Instructor Evaluation	Comments
9. Rinse patient's mouth to ensure all etchant is removed from tooth surface (thirty seconds).			3		
10. Dry tooth or teeth (will have chalky appearance).			3		
11. Prepare bonding agent according to manufacturer's directions.			3		
12. Apply bonding to back of bracket.			3		
13. Pass the agent to the dentist for placement on tooth.			3		
14. Bracket is passed and orthodontist positions it on the tooth.			3		
15. Excess bonding agent is removed with a scaler or similar instrument from around bracket.			3		
16. Brackets are held in position on tooth until bonding material is set chemically or with curing light.			3		
17. Remove the cotton rolls.			2		
18. Remove the retractors from patient's mouth.			2		

TOTAL POINTS POSSIBLE   82

TOTAL POINTS POSSIBLE—2nd Attempt   80

TOTAL POINTS EARNED   _____

Points assigned reflect importance of step to meeting objective: Important = 1; Essential = 2; Critical = 3. Students will lose 2 points for repeated attempts. Failure results if any of the critical steps are omitted or performed incorrectly. If using a 100-point scale, determine score by dividing points earned by total points possible and multiplying the results by 100.

SCORE: _____

SKILL COMPETENCY ASSESSMENT

21-4 Placement of the Arch Wire and Ligature Ties
(corresponds to textbook Procedure 21-6)

Student's Name _____ Date _____

Instructor's Name _____

SKILL   Routine steps should be followed for all treatment areas to maintain absolute clinical asepsis. The dental assistant must be prepared and thinking ahead to anticipate the dentist's needs. The orthodontist selects and shapes the arch wire so that once the bands and brackets are placed, the arch wire can be positioned and secured in place. The arch wire is commonly secured into the brackets with elastic or stainless steel ligatures (ties) and/or slot Damon SL.

PERFORMANCE OBJECTIVE   The student will follow a routine procedure that meets the regulations and the protocol set forth by the dentist and regulatory agencies, keeping in mind that assistants' duties vary from state to state. The assistant may be evaluated by performance, statement, and/or combined responses and action.

	Self Evaluation	Student Evaluation	Possible Points	Instructor Evaluation	Comments
Equipment and Supplies					
1. Basic setup: mouth mirror, explorer, and cotton pliers			3		
2. Cotton rolls and gauze			3		
3. Saliva ejector and HVE			3		
4. Selected arch wire			3		
5. Weingart pliers			3		
6. Bird beak pliers			3		
7. Elastics or ligature wire			3		
8. Ligature cutting pliers			3		
9. Ligature tying pliers			3		
10. Distal-end cutting pliers			3		
11. Condenser			3		
Competency Steps					
1. Insert arch wire into buccal tubes on molar bands using Weingart pliers.			3		
2. If wire is too long, cut ends off with distal-end cutting pliers.			3		
3. Arch wire is placed in brackets' horizontal slots along the arch.			3		
A. Elastic ties			3		
B. Ligature wire			3		
C. Damon SL bracket			3		
Elastic Ties Placement					
1. This method is to secure the arch wire in brackets with elastic ties.			3		
2. Ties are spread and placed on gingival extensions of brackets.			3		

21-4 continued *(corresponds to textbook Procedure 21-6)*

	Self Evaluation	Student Evaluation	Possible Points	Instructor Evaluation	Comments
3. Tie is pulled over the arch wire.			3		
4. Tie is wrapped around the occlusal extensions of the brackets.			3		
Ligature Wire Ties Placement					
1. Hold ligature wire between thumb and the index finger.			3		
2. Wrap wire around the occlusal and gingival wings of bracket in distal-mesial direction.			3		
3. Cross ends of wire together.			3		
4. Using a hemostat or ligature tying pliers, twist ends of the wire together for several rotations.			3		
5. Repeat process to secure the arch wire.			3		
6. Twisted ends of ligature wire, called the "pigtail," are cut with ligature wire cutting pliers 3 to 4 mm.			3		
7. Pigtail is bent into embrasure space with condenser.			3		
8. When all pigtail ends have been tucked into place, run finger over the area to check for sharp ends.			3		
9. Check distal ends of arch wire. Cut any excess with distal-end cutting pliers.			3		
Rubber Elastic Bands					
1. Patient is shown how to place and remove them.			3		
2. Instructions are given on how often to change the rubber bands.			3		
3. Patient is given a sufficient number of bands with instructions to call the office for more, if needed.			3		

TOTAL POINTS POSSIBLE   99

TOTAL POINTS POSSIBLE—2nd Attempt   97

TOTAL POINTS EARNED   _____

Points assigned reflect importance of step to meeting objective: Important = 1; Essential = 2; Critical = 3. Students will lose 2 points for repeated attempts. Failure results if any of the critical steps are omitted or performed incorrectly. If using a 100-point scale, determine score by dividing points earned by total points possible and multiplying the results by 100.

SCORE: _____

SKILL COMPETENCY ASSESSMENT

21-5 Completion Appointment *(corresponds to textbook Procedure 21-7)*

Student's Name _____ Date _____

Instructor's Name _____

SKILL Routine steps should be followed for all treatment areas to maintain absolute clinical asepsis. The dental assistant must be prepared and thinking ahead to anticipate the dentist's needs. Once the teeth have moved into the position and the orthodontist is satisfied with the treatment, the braces are removed. The patient receives a coronal polish and an impression is taken for use in construction of a retainer or positioner to hold the teeth in position for the alveolar bone to stabilize the new position of the teeth.

PERFORMANCE OBJECTIVE The student will follow a routine procedure that meets the regulations and the protocol set forth by the dentist and regulatory agencies, keeping in mind that assistants' duties vary from state to state. The assistant may be evaluated by performance, statement, and/or combined responses and action. When the orthodontist determines the patient's teeth have moved to the desired position, the appliances are removed.

	Self Evaluation	Student Evaluation	Possible Points	Instructor Evaluation	Comments
Equipment and Supplies					
1. Basic setup: mouth mirror, explorer, and cotton pliers			3		
2. Cotton rolls and gauze			3		
3. Scaler			3		
4. Ligature wire cutting pliers			3		
5. Hemostat			3		
6. Bracket and adhesive removing pliers			3		
7. Posterior band remover			3		
8. Ultrasonic scaler (optional)			3		
9. Prophy angle, cups, and prophy paste			3		
10. Alginate impression material and selected tray			3		
Competency Steps					
1. Ligature ties are loosened with a scaler or explorer.			3		
2. Cut ligature with wire cutting pliers.			3		
Elastic Bands					
1. Elastic ties are removed with a scaler.			3		
2. Scaler is placed under elastic.			3		
3. Roll elastic over the bracket wings until elastic is released.			3		
Ligature Wire Ties					
1. Place beaks of ligature wire cutting pliers where wire is exposed.			3		
2. Cut the wire.			3		
3. Carefully remove the wire from the wings of the bracket.			3		
4. Repeat on each tooth until all ligature wires are removed.			3		

21-5 continued *(corresponds to textbook Procedure 21-7)*

	Self Evaluation	Student Evaluation	Possible Points	Instructor Evaluation	Comments
5. Using a hemostat, remove the arch wire from the brackets.			3		
6. Pull arch wire from the buccal tube on one side.			3		
7. Hold the arch wire securely to prevent injury to patient while removing the opposite end.			3		
Anterior Bracket Removal					
1. Use a bracket and adhesive-removal pliers.			3		
A. Place lower beak of pliers from the gingival edge of the bracket.			3		
B. Place nylon tip of pliers on occlusal edge of bracket.			3		
2. Pliers are squeezed together and breaks bond and removes some cement.			3		
Posterior Band Removal					
1. Band-removing pliers are placed with the cushioned end on buccal cusp.			3		
2. Blade end of the pliers is placed against the gingival edge of the band.			3		
3. Band is gently lifted toward the occlusal surface.			3		
4. This process is repeated on the lingual surface until the band is free.			3		
Completion Phase					
1. Cement and direct bonding materials are removed from tooth surfaces with a hand scaler, an ultrasonic scaler, and/or a finishing bur.			3		
2. A rubber cup polish is completed.			3		
3. Photographs may be taken.			2		
4. An alginate impression is taken of both arches.			3		
5. Impressions are sent to the lab for construction of the retainer.			2		
6. Patient is reappointed for later that day or next.			3		
7. Retainer or positioner is placed.			3		
8. Patient is given instruction on placement and removal of the removable appliance and the wearing schedule.			3		

TOTAL POINTS POSSIBLE   112

TOTAL POINTS POSSIBLE—2nd Attempt   110

TOTAL POINTS EARNED   _____

Points assigned reflect importance of step to meeting objective: Important = 1; Essential = 2; Critical = 3. Students will lose 2 points for repeated attempts. Failure results if any of the critical steps are omitted or performed incorrectly. If using a 100-point scale, determine score by dividing points earned by total points possible and multiplying the results by 100.

SCORE: _____

CHAPTER 22

Pediatric Dentistry

OBJECTIVES

The student should strive to meet the following objectives and demonstrate an understanding of the facts and principles presented in this chapter:

1. Define pediatric dentistry as a specialty.
2. Describe the pediatric office and team members.
3. Explain common behavior characteristics of children of various ages.
4. Describe child behavior management techniques.
5. Explain the role of the parent or guardian in pediatric dentistry.
6. Identify common procedures in pediatric dentistry.
7. Identify the equipment unique to pediatric dentistry.
8. Explain common emergencies in pediatric dentistry and the treatment for these emergencies.
9. Identify the signs of child abuse and the procedure for reporting suspected child abuse cases.

SUMMARY

The scope of the pediatric treatment for the child patient includes restoring and maintaining the primary, mixed, and permanent dentition and applying preventive measures for dental caries, periodontal disease, and malocclusion. The primary focus of the pediatric dental practice is preventive treatment and dealing with the compromised child patient. The whole staff needs to enjoy working with children and be sincere and honest in their actions and feelings. To be effective in the management of children, the dental team must keep upbeat, motivated, and aware.

The role of the dental assistant in the pediatric practice will vary depending on areas of responsibility. One aspect is the management of the child. Another is the work at chairside. Skills the assistant performs at chairside vary in every office and from state to state depending on the state Dental Practice Act. When the assistant works independently, he or she assumes the authority role and must maintain control of the child. The dental assistant is also an educator, both with the child and the parents.

KEY TERMS

apexogenesis
avulsed tooth
behavior management
direct pulp capping (DPC)
fluoride applications
hand-over-mouth (HOM)
   technique
indirect pulp treatment (IPT)
maturation

modeling technique
mouth guards
objective fears
open bay
pedodontics
pit and fissure sealants
pulpectomy
pulpotomy

space maintainers
spot-welded matrix bands
stainless steel crowns
subjective fears
T-band matrix
tell, show, and do technique
tongue thrust
traumatic intrusion

EXERCISES AND ACTIVITIES

1. What specialty practice provides dental care for children and the compromised child patient? _____
   A. Orthodontics
   C. Endodontics
   B. Pedodontics
   D. General dentistry

2. What treatment area is designed with several chairs arranged in one open area? _____
   A. Quiet room
   B. Prevention room
   C. Open bay
   D. Reading room

3. The best age to introduce dental care in the dental office is _____
   A. two to six.
   B. One to two.
   C. Infant to one.
   D. None of the above

4. Fear is a large factor in behavior problems with children. Objective fears are based on _____
   A. suggestions from others.
   B. attitudes from others.
   C. concerns developed from others.
   D. the child's own experience.

5. There are a variety of behavior management techniques. If the child is told the name of the instrument, the assistant demonstrates it, and the instrument is used, this is called _____
   A. voice control.
   B. tell, show, do.
   C. subjective.
   D. nonverbal.

6. One behavior management technique pairs a timid child in dental chair with a cooperative child of similar age. This process is called _____
   A. positive reinforcement.
   B. distraction.
   C. modeling.
   D. nonverbal communication.

7. Children that are actively involved in contact sports should be fitted for a _____
   A. fixed space maintainer.
   B. removable space maintainer.
   C. dental matrix.
   D. mouth guard.

8. Behavior modification is sometimes necessary. Fixed appliances such as cribs and rakes are used to prevent what oral habit? _____
   A. Thumb sucking
   B. Tongue thrust
   C. Modeling
   D. Pulpotomy

9. What custom matrix is designed and used on primary teeth? _____
   A. T-band
   B. Tofflemire
   C. Space maintainer
   D. Stainless steel crown

10. What custom-made matrix bands are used on primary teeth for Class II restorations? _____
    A. T-band
    B. Tofflemire
    C. Spot-welded
    D. Stainless steel crown

11. If the pulp has been exposed through mechanical or traumatic means, but there is a chance for a favorable response, what procedure is indicated? _____
    A. Direct pulp capping
    B. Pulpotomy
    C. Apexogenesis
    D. Pulpectomy

12. If the pulp of a primary or young permanent tooth has been exposed, what procedure may be indicated to remove a portion of the pulp? _____
    A. Direct pulp capping
    B. Pulpotomy
    C. Apexogenesis
    D. Pulpectomy

13. For the young permanent teeth, a pulpotomy maintains the pulp vitality and allows enough time for the root end to develop and close. In these cases, the treatment is called _____
    A. direct pulp capping.
    B. pulpectomy.
    C. apexogenesis.
    D. avulsed.

14. What procedure involves the complete removal of the dental pulp? _____
    A. Pulpectomy   C. Pulpotomy
    B. Apexogenesis   D. Pulp capping

15. What condition occurs when the teeth are forcibly driven into the alveolus so that only a portion of the crown is visible? _____
    A. Displaced tooth
    B. Avulsed tooth
    C. Traumatic intrusion
    D. Apexogenesis

16. When a tooth has been completely removed from the mouth, it is termed _____
    A. displaced.
    B. traumatic intrusion.
    C. apexogenesis.
    D. avulsed.

17. Dentists should report suspicious signs of child abuse to a _____
    A. social service agency.
    B. local police department.
    C. child protective service.
    D. All of the above

18. The following general behavior characteristics fit children of what age? _____
    1. Can respond to the dentist's instructions
    2. Can understand simple explanations
    3. Like to be with parents and siblings
    4. Like to play—see the "squirt gun," for example

    A. Four to six
    B. Two to six
    C. Two to four
    D. Six to twelve

SKILL COMPETENCY ASSESSMENT

22-1 T-Band Placement

Student's Name _____ Date _____

Instructor's Name _____

SKILL   Routine steps should be followed for all treatment areas to maintain absolute clinical asepsis. The dental assistant must be prepared and thinking ahead to anticipate the dentist's needs. T-bands are designed and used on primary teeth. They come in various designs and sizes. They are often made of brass strips that are "crossed" at one end. The T-bands do not require a retainer, are adjustable, and can be secured on the tooth.

PERFORMANCE OBJECTIVE   The student will follow a routine procedure that meets the regulations and the protocol set forth by the dentist and regulatory agencies, keeping in mind that assistants' duties vary from state to state. The assistant may be evaluated by performance, statement, and/or combined responses and action. For this procedure, the tooth has been prepared and matrix is assembled and placed on the tooth.

	Self Evaluation	Student Evaluation	Possible Points	Instructor Evaluation	Comments
Equipment and Supplies					
1. T-band assortment			3		
2. Burnisher			3		
3. Cotton pliers or hemostat			3		
4. Crown and collar scissors			3		
Competency Steps					
1. Select appropriate size T-band (can be done ahead).			3		
2. Band is looped to shape approximate diameter of tooth.			3		
3. The "T" ends are folded over band loop, leaving a circle with long tail or end.			3		
4. Band is placed on tooth, into interproximal space covering the margins of preparation.			3		
5. Where the "T" is folded is placed on the buccal surface, away from the margins of the preparation.			3		
6. Band is tightened by pulling on free end (tail) until band is tight around the tooth.			3		
7. Free end is bent back toward the "T" to secure band.			3		
8. The excess band is removed with scissors.			3		
9. The band is wedged and burnished.			3		
10. To remove the T-band, fold back the overlapping section of band to loosen the band.			3		

22-1 continued

	Self Evaluation	Student Evaluation	Possible Points	Instructor Evaluation	Comments
11. Use cotton pliers to remove band from tooth.			3		

TOTAL POINTS POSSIBLE	45	
TOTAL POINTS POSSIBLE—2nd Attempt	43	
TOTAL POINTS EARNED	_____	

Points assigned reflect importance of step to meeting objective: Important = 1; Essential = 2; Critical = 3. Students will lose 2 points for repeated attempts. Failure results if any of the critical steps are omitted or performed incorrectly. If using a 100-point scale, determine score by dividing points earned by total points possible and multiplying the results by 100.

SCORE: _____

SKILL COMPETENCY ASSESSMENT

22-2 Pulpotomy *(corresponds to textbook Procedure 22-3)*

Student's Name _____ Date _____

Instructor's Name _____

SKILL Routine steps should be followed for all treatment areas to maintain absolute clinical asepsis. The dental assistant must be prepared and thinking ahead to anticipate the dentist's needs.

PERFORMANCE OBJECTIVE The student will follow a routine procedure that meets the regulations and the protocol set forth by the dentist and regulatory agencies, keeping in mind that assistants' duties vary from state to state. The dental assistant prepares the treatment room, patient, equipment, and supplies. The tooth is opened and treated before a temporary restoration is placed. The assistant may be evaluated by performance, statement, and/or combined responses and action.

	Self Evaluation	Student Evaluation	Possible Points	Instructor Evaluation	Comments
Equipment and Supplies					
1. Amalgam setup			3		
2. Formocresol			3		
3. Sterile round burs			3		
4. Zinc oxide-eugenol cement (ZOE or IRM)			3		
Competency Steps					
1. Anesthetic administered.			2		
2. Place dental dam.			3		
3. High-speed handpiece with bur in place.			3		
4. Coronal portion of pulp removed with spoon excavator or round bur.			3		
5. Prepare sterile cotton pellet, wetting it with formocresol.			3		
6. Pass pellet to dentist for placement in chamber for five minutes.			3		
7. After the hemorrhage is controlled, the cotton pellet is removed and the pulp chamber is rinsed and dried.			3		
8. Mix zinc oxide-eugenol to base consistency.			3		
9. Pass the base to the dentist.			3		
10. Place restoration of choice, such as amalgam.			3		
11. Remove rubber dam.			3		
12. Check occlusion.			3		

22-2 continued *(corresponds to textbook Procedure 22-3)*

	Self Evaluation	Student Evaluation	Possible Points	Instructor Evaluation	Comments
13. Options to amalgam (stainless steel crown and/or temporary restoration).			3		
TOTAL POINTS POSSIBLE			50		
TOTAL POINTS POSSIBLE—2nd Attempt			48		
TOTAL POINTS EARNED			_____		

Points assigned reflect importance of step to meeting objective: Important = 1; Essential = 2; Critical = 3. Students will lose 2 points for repeated attempts. Failure results if any of the critical steps are omitted or performed incorrectly. If using a 100-point scale, determine score by dividing points earned by total points possible and multiplying the results by 100.

SCORE: _____

Periodontics

OBJECTIVES

The student should strive to meet the following objectives and demonstrate an understanding of the facts and principles presented in this chapter:

1. Describe the scope of periodontics.
2. Identify members of the periodontal team and their roles.
3. Describe the stages of periodontal disease.
4. Explain the diagnostic procedure involved in the patient's first visit to the periodontal office.
5. Identify and describe periodontal instruments and their uses.
6. Describe non-surgical procedures and the dental assistant's role in each procedure.
7. Explain surgical procedures and dental assisting responsibilities.
8. Identify the types of periodontal dressing and how they are prepared, placed, and removed.
9. Describe periodontal maintenance procedures and the patient's role relating to each.

SUMMARY

Periodontal disease is as old as the human race. According to the American Academy of Periodontology, three out of four adults will experience, to some degree, periodontal problems at some time in their lives. Periodontal disease occurs in children and adolescents with marginal gingivitis and gingival recession, the most prevalent conditions.

The dental assistant performs chairside assisting duties and the expanded functions allowed by the state Dental Practice Act, including placing and removing periodontal dressing, removing sutures, and performing coronal polishes. The dental assistant takes radiographs, makes impressions for study models, places sealants, and administers fluoride treatments. The assistant also gives pre- and postoperative instructions and prepares the treatment room for surgery. These functions are in addition to treatment room preparation and maintenance and sterilization procedures. The dental assistant is involved in educating and motivating the patient throughout the treatment. In some offices, the dental assistant may also perform laboratory tasks, such as pouring study models or making periodontal splints.

KEY TERMS

bone resorption	gingivitis	periodontal flap surgery	pocket marking pliers
bruxism	gingivoplasty	periodontal knives	prophylaxis
calculus	hoe scaler	periodontal pocket	recession
coronal polish	interdental knives	periodontal probe	root planing
curette	mucogingival surgery	periodontal probing	scaling
electrosurgery	occlusal equilibration	periodontitis	sickle scalers
frenectomy	osseous surgery	periodontium	surgical scalpel
furcation	ostectomy	periosteal elevators	tooth mobility
gingival grafting	osteoplasty	plaque	ultrasonic instruments
gingivectomy	periodontal dressing		

EXERCISES AND ACTIVITIES

1. Bacterial plaque forms around the margin of the gingiva and, if left undisturbed, it will mineralize and appear as a yellow or brown deposit on the teeth called _____
   A. food.
   B. plaque.
   C. calculus.
   D. a stain.

2. Grinding of the teeth is called _____
   A. mobility.
   B. pockets.
   C. bruxism.
   D. resorption.

3. A curved instrument is used to measure destruction of the interradicular bone of multi-rooted teeth. Name the area where the roots divide. _____
   A. Sulcus
   B. Furcation
   C. Mesiofacial
   D. Distofacial

4. During the periodontal exam, the gingival tissue is measured with a periodontal probe to evaluate _____
   A. plaque.
   B. calculus.
   C. mobility.
   D. recession.

5. What calibrated instrument is used to measure the depth of periodontal pockets? _____
   A. Curette
   B. Periodontal knives
   C. Periodontal hoe
   D. Periodontal probe

6. What hand instrument is used to remove hard deposits of supragingival and subgingival calculus from teeth. The working end has two sharp edges that come to a point. _____
   A. Sickle scaler
   B. Periodontal hoe
   C. Orban knives
   D. Curette

7. What hand instrument's working end has a cutting edge on one or both sides of the blade and the end is rounded? It is used primarily for removing subgingival calculus. _____
   A. Sickle scaler
   B. Periodontal hoe
   C. Orban knives
   D. Curette

8. What hand instrument's cutting edge has a blade bent at a 90° angle at the end of the working end and is beveled? _____
   A. Chisel scaler
   B. Gracey curette
   C. Hoe scaler
   D. Universal curette

9. These periodontal knives or gingivectomy knives are used to remove gingival tissue during periodontal surgery. The common shape is broad bladed. _____
   A. Orban
   B. Scalpel
   C. Kirkland
   D. Pocket marking pliers

10. The interdental knives that are used to remove soft tissue interproximally and whose blades are long and narrow are called _____
    A. Orban.
    B. scalpels.
    C. Kirkland.
    D. pocket marking pliers.

11. What fast and effective instrument can be used as an adjunct to manual scaling procedures? The water spray cools and flushes the area. _____
    A. Electrosurgery unit
    B. Ultrasonic unit
    C. Surgical scalpel
    D. Universal curette

12. What instrument is used to coagulate blood during the incisure of gingival tissue? _____
    A. Ultrasonic unit
    B. Electrosurgery unit
    C. Universal curette
    D. Gracey curette

13. When the beaks of the _____ are pinched together, the gingival tissue is perforated, leaving small pinpoint markings.
    A. periodontal probe
    B. pocket marking pliers
    C. cotton forceps
    D. periosteal elevator

14. What instrument is used to reflect soft tissue away from the bone? _____
    A. Periodontal probe
    B. Pocket marking pliers
    C. Curette
    D. Periosteal elevator

15. In a routine _____, deposits above and below the gingival margins are removed, and the coronal surfaces of the teeth are polished with rubber cups and brushes.
    A. root planing
    B. curettage
    C. prophylaxis
    D. scaling

16. _____ is the process of planing or shaving the root surface to leave a smooth root surface.
    A. Root planing
    B. Curettage
    C. Osteoplasty
    D. Ostectomy

17. The process that involves reshaping the gingival tissue to remove deformities is _____
    A. gingivectomy.   C. frenectomy.
    B. gingivoplasty.   D. mucogingival surgery.

18. Periodontal flap surgery involves surgically separating the _____ from the underlying tissue.
    A. bone   C. gingiva
    B. tooth   D. sulcus

19. This surgery is reconstructive surgery on the gingiva and/or mucosa tissues. _____
    A. Frenectomy   C. Gingival grafting
    B. Mucogingival   D. Ostectomy

20. What procedure involves taking tissue from one site and placing it on another? _____
    A. Frenectomy
    B. Mucogingival surgery
    C. Gingival grafting
    D. Ostectomy

21. What procedure is a complete removal of the frenum, including the attachment to the underlying bone? _____
    A. Frenectomy
    B. Mucogingival surgery
    C. Gingival grafting
    D. Ostectomy

22. The periodontium includes which of the following? _____
    1. Calculus
    2. Food
    3. Debris
    4. Sulcus
    5. Gingiva
    6. Epithelial attachment
    7. Bone
    8. Plaque

    A. 1, 2, 3, 8
    B. 4, 5, 6, 7
    C. 2, 3, 4, 8
    D. 2, 3, 5, 6

23. Causes and indications of gingivitis include which of the following? _____
    1. Plaque buildup
    2. Calculus buildup
    3. Periodontal pocket
    4. Loose teeth (mobility)
    5. Tissues reddish in color
    6. Halitosis

    A. 1, 2, 5
    B. 3, 4, 6
    C. 1, 2, 3
    D. 2, 3, 6

24. When margins of the gingiva and periodontal fibers recede and the supporting bone becomes inflamed and destroyed, this condition is called _____
    A. gingivitis.   B. periodontitis.

25. When tissues become reddish in color, interdental papilla may be swollen and bulbous, and tissues may bleed after brushing and flossing, this condition is called _____
    A. gingivitis.   B. periodontitis.

26. Periodontal probing is measuring the depth of the periodontal pocket with a periodontal probe. Each tooth will have _____ sites probed and recorded.
    A. three   B. six

27. What surgical procedure reduces the height of the gingival tissue by removal of diseased gingival tissue that forms the periodontal pocket? _____
    A. Gingivoplasty   B. Gingivectomy

28. What procedure reshapes the gingival tissue to remove deformities such as clefts, craters, and enlargements? _____
    A. Gingivoplasty   B. Gingivectomy

29. What type of osseous surgery reshapes the bone? _____
    A. Osteoplasty   B. Ostectomy

30. What type of osseous surgery removes bone? _____
    A. Osteoplasty   B. Ostectomy

SKILL COMPETENCY ASSESSMENT

| 23-1 Scaling, Curettage, and Polishing *(corresponds to textbook Procedure 23-2)*

Student's Name _____ Date _____

Instructor's Name _____

SKILL The purpose of scaling is to remove plaque, calculus, and stains from the surfaces of the teeth. Gingival curettage, also known as soft tissue curettage, is a procedure that involves the scraping of the inner gingival walls of the periodontal pockets to remove inflamed tissue and debris. The deposits above the gingival margin, supragingival deposits, and those just below the gingival margin, subgingival, are removed with scalers and curettes. After this, the coronal surfaces of the teeth are polished with rubber cups, brushes, an abrasive, porte polishers, and dental tape. Depending on the state Dental Practice Act, dental assistants can remove supragingival deposits and/or perform the coronal polish. The dental assistant must be prepared and thinking ahead to anticipate the dentist's and/or dental hygienist's needs. Routine steps should be followed for all treatment areas to maintain absolute clinical asepsis.

PERFORMANCE OBJECTIVE The student will follow a routine procedure that meets the regulations and the protocol set forth by the dentist and regulatory agencies, keeping in mind that assistants' duties vary from state to state. The assistant may be evaluated by performance, statement, and/or combined responses and action. The procedure is done by the dentist or the dental hygienist. A dental hygiene assistant assists during this procedure; responsibilities include instrument transfer, rinsing the oral cavity, evacuation with the HVE, removing debris from instruments, retraction, and patient comfort.

	Self Evaluation	Student Evaluation	Possible Points	Instructor Evaluation	Comments
Equipment and Supplies					
1. Basic setup: mouth mirror, explorer, cotton pliers			3		
2. Cotton rolls and 2 x 2 gauze sponges			2		
3. Saliva ejector, HVE tip, air-water syringe tip			3		
4. Periodontal probe			3		
5. Scalers: Jacque and Shepherd's hook			3		
6. Curettes: Universal and Gracey			3		
7. Dental floss and dental tape			3		
8. Prophy angle—rubber cups and brushes			3		
9. Prophy paste			2		
10. Optional—disclosing solution or tablets					
Competency Steps					
1. The operator examines the oral cavity.			3		
2. Operator uses scalers and curettes to remove calculus and debris from around teeth (operator cleans all surfaces of teeth in one quadrant before moving to next quadrant).			3		
3. Keep area clean and clear with HVE and air-water as directed.			3		
4. Transfer instruments as directed.			3		
5. Operator polishes teeth with prophy paste, rubber cup, and brush. Some practices use a prophy jet spray (spray salt water) as an alternative to rubber cup polish.			3		

23-1 continued (corresponds to textbook Procedure 23-2)

	Self Evaluation	Student Evaluation	Possible Points	Instructor Evaluation	Comments
6. Operator uses dental tape and prophy paste to clean interproximal areas.			3		
7. The entire mouth is flossed and rinsed.			3		

TOTAL POINTS POSSIBLE   46

TOTAL POINTS POSSIBLE—2nd Attempt   44

TOTAL POINTS EARNED   _____

Points assigned reflect importance of step to meeting objective: Important = 1; Essential = 2; Critical = 3. Students will lose 2 points for repeated attempts. Failure results if any of the critical steps are omitted or performed incorrectly. If using a 100-point scale, determine score by dividing points earned by total points possible and multiplying the results by 100.

SCORE: _____

SKILL COMPETENCY ASSESSMENT

23-2 Gingivectomy (corresponds to textbook Procedure 23-3)

Student's Name _____ Date _____

Instructor's Name _____

SKILL This surgical procedure reduces the height of the gingival tissue, which provides visibility and access to remove irritants and smooth the root surface.

Depending on the state Dental Practice Act, dental assistants may place and remove the periodontal dressing. The dental assistant must be prepared and thinking ahead to anticipate the dentist's needs. Routine steps should be followed for all treatment areas to maintain absolute clinical asepsis.

PERFORMANCE OBJECTIVE The student will follow a routine procedure that meets the regulations and the protocol set forth by the dentist and regulatory agencies, keeping in mind that assistants' duties vary from state to state. The assistant may be evaluated by performance, statement, and/or combined responses and action. The procedure is done by the periodontist to remove disease gingiva and clean the periodontal pockets. The dental assistant prepares the instruments and materials, prepares the patient, and performs assisting responsibilities during the procedure. According to state Dental Practice Acts, the dental assistant may place and remove the periodontal dressing.

	Self Evaluation	Student Evaluation	Possible Points	Instructor Evaluation	Comments
Equipment and Supplies					
1. Basic setup: mouth mirror, explorer, cotton pliers			3		
2. Cotton rolls and 2 x 2 gauze sponges			2		
3. Saliva ejector, HVE tip, air-water syringe tip, surgical aspirator tip			3		
4. Periodontal probe			3		
5. Anesthetic setup			3		
6. Pocket marker			3		
7. Periodontal knives—broad bladed and interproximal			3		
8. Scalpel, blades, and diamond burs			3		
9. Scalers and curettes			3		
10. Soft tissue rongeurs and surgical scissors			3		
11. Hemostat			3		
12. Suture needle and thread			3		
13. Periodontal dressing materials			3		
Competency Steps					
1. Anesthetic is administered to anesthetize tissues and reduce blood flow to area.			3		
2. Area examined with periodontal probe.			3		
3. The depths of pockets are marked with pocket marker.			3		
4. Transfer instruments as directed.			3		
5. The broad-bladed knife or scalpel is used to incise the marked gingiva area.			3		

23-2 continued (corresponds to textbook Procedure 23-3)

	Self Evaluation	Student Evaluation	Possible Points	Instructor Evaluation	Comments
6. Evacuate the area and transfer instruments.			3		
7. Interdental knives are used to remove interproximal tissue.			3		
8. Scissors, rongeurs, and burs are used to remove tissue tags.			3		
9. Have gauze ready to receive any tissue from instruments and to clean the area of debris.			3		
10. After tissue is removed, periodontist scales and planes the root surface.			3		
11. Continue to pass instruments and evacuate the area.			3		
12. Sterile saline solution may be used to irrigate.			2		
13. If sutures are needed, prepare suture needle and thread and position in a hemostat.			3		
14. Pass the hemostat and transfer scissors as needed.			3		
15. Retract tissue as needed.			3		
16. After sutures are placed, area is irrigated with sterile saline solution.			3		
17. Evacuate the area.			3		
18. Prepare the periodontal dressing.			3		
19. Assist the dentist with periodontal dressing placement.			3		
20. Give the patient postoperative instructions.			3		
21. Make sure patient does not have any debris on his or her face.			2		
22. Patient is dismissed.			2		

TOTAL POINTS POSSIBLE   101

TOTAL POINTS POSSIBLE—2nd Attempt   99

TOTAL POINTS EARNED   _____

Points assigned reflect importance of step to meeting objective: Important = 1; Essential = 2; Critical = 3. Students will lose 2 points for repeated attempts. Failure results if any of the critical steps are omitted or performed incorrectly. If using a 100-point scale, determine score by dividing points earned by total points possible and multiplying the results by 100.

SCORE: _____

SKILL COMPETENCY ASSESSMENT

23-3 Preparation and Placement of the Non-Eugenol Periodontal Dressing
(corresponds to textbook Procedure 23-5)

Student's Name _____ Date _____

Instructor's Name _____

SKILL Periodontal dressing or packs are placed after periodontal surgical procedures. The dressing does not have any medicinal qualities but acts like a bandage to protect the tissue during the healing process. There are different materials used for periodontal dressing. The most common types are the zinc oxide-eugenol materials and the non-eugenol materials.

The dental assistant must be prepared and thinking ahead to anticipate the dentist's needs. Routine steps should be followed for all treatment areas to maintain absolute clinical asepsis.

PERFORMANCE OBJECTIVE The student will follow a routine procedure that meets the regulations and the protocol set forth by the dentist and regulatory agencies, keeping in mind that assistants' duties vary from state to state. The assistant may be evaluated by performance, statement, and/or combined responses and action. The dentist routinely places the dressing, but in some states the dental assistant is allowed to place and remove the periodontal dressing. The dressing is placed after the surgery to protect the tissues and promote the healing process.

	Self Evaluation	Student Evaluation	Possible Points	Instructor Evaluation	Comments
Equipment and Supplies					
1. Basic setup: mouth mirror, explorer, and cotton pliers			3		
2. Gauze sponges			2		
3. Non-eugenol periodontal dressing material (base and accelerator)			3		
4. Paper pad and tongue depressor			3		
5. Lubricant			3		
6. Instrument to contour dressing (spoon excavator, sickle scaler)			3		
Competency Steps					
1. Patient's lips are lightly coated with Vaseline (after the hemorrhaging is controlled).			3		
2. Dressing materials are dispensed into equal lengths.			3		
3. Dressing materials are mixed with a tongue blade until homogeneous.			3		
4. Material is allowed to set for two to three minutes or until tackiness is gone.			3		
5. Lubricate gloved fingers with Vaseline so the putty-like material can be easily handled.			3		
6. Dressing comes with a retardant to slow setting time, if necessary; molded easily for three to five minutes and worked for fifteen to twenty.			3		
7. Dressing is molded into a thin strip slightly longer than length of surgical site.			3		
8. Divide strip into two equal lengths, one for facial surface and one for lingual surface.			3		
9. Begin placement; form end of one strip into a hook shape.			3		

23-3 continued *(corresponds to textbook Procedure 23-5)*

	Self Evaluation	Student Evaluation	Possible Points	Instructor Evaluation	Comments
10. Wrap hook around the distal of the most posterior tooth.			3		
11. Adapt the rest of strip along facial surface, gently pressing pack into interproximal areas.			3		
12. Second strip is applied to lingual surface in same manner. Pack is wrapped around the last posterior tooth and adapted to lingual surface, moving toward the midline.			3		
13. Pack should cover the gingiva evenly without interfering with occlusion or tongue movement.			3		
14. Check dressing for overextensions.			3		
15. Excess dressing is removed with a spoon excavator or scaler.			3		
16. Gently press instrument into dressing to detach extra material.			3		
17. Smooth pack and evaluate for even thickness.			3		
18. Ask patient how pack feels.			2		
19. Patient can move tongue, cheeks, and lips to mold pack.			2		
20. Make adjustments, ensure dressing is securely in place, trimmed, and contoured.			3		
21. Give patient instructions:					
A. Pack is kept on for one week after surgery			2		
B. Pack will harden in a few hours and withstand normal chewing stresses			2		
C. Pack may chip and break off during week but should remain intact as long as possible			2		
D. If pain when pieces of pack come off or becomes rough, patient should call office			2		
E. Patient should brush the occlusal surface of teeth involved in surgery			2		
F. Continue to brush and floss rest of teeth as normal			2		

TOTAL POINTS POSSIBLE	87	
TOTAL POINTS POSSIBLE—2nd Attempt	85	
TOTAL POINTS EARNED	_____	

Points assigned reflect importance of step to meeting objective: Important = 1; Essential = 2; Critical = 3. Students will lose 2 points for repeated attempts. Failure results if any of the critical steps are omitted or performed incorrectly. If using a 100-point scale, determine score by dividing points earned by total points possible and multiplying the results by 100.

SCORE: _____

Fixed Prosthodontics

The student should strive to meet the following objectives and demonstrate an understanding of the facts and principles presented in this chapter:

1. Define the scope of fixed prosthodontics.
2. Explain considerations the dentist must make when recommending various prostheses to a patient.
3. Describe various types of fixed prostheses and their functions.
4. Describe dental materials used in fixed prostheses.
5. Explain the involvement of the laboratory technician in the fabrication of fixed prostheses.
6. Describe the role of the dental assistant in all phases of fixed prosthodontic treatment.
7. Explain techniques for retaining the prosthesis when there is little or no crown on the tooth.
8. Describe implant retainer prostheses.
9. Explain techniques for maintaining fixed prostheses.

SUMMARY

Fixed prosthodontics is the specialty that deals with replacement of missing teeth or parts of teeth with extensive restorations. There are many types of fixed prostheses and a variety of materials used for preparation, fabrication, and cementation. The dental assistant is very involved in all stages of fixed prosthodontic treatment. It is important to understand the sequence of the procedure and the different types of restorations when assisting the dentist.

The goal of this chapter is to assess the more common procedures to give the dental assistant the background and sequence to assist the dentist. The restorations routinely take at least two appointments to complete. The assistant explains the steps of the procedure to the patient, answers questions, and gives postoperative and home care instructions.

KEY TERMS

abutments	Maryland bridge	prostheses
bite registration	onlays	retention core
dental casting alloy	partial crown	retention pins
fixed prosthetic	pontic	shade guide
full-cast crown	porcelain-fused-to-metal crowns	veneers
inlays	post-retained cores	

EXERCISES AND ACTIVITIES

1. Replacing missing teeth will benefit the patient by _____
    A. restoring masticatory function.
    B. improving esthetics.
    C. improving speech.
    D. preventing further movement of teeth.
    E. All of the above

2. The artificial part replacing a missing tooth is called a _____
    A. retention pin.
    B. retention core.
    C. retention post.
    D. prosthesis.

3. A(n) _____ covers the entire coronal surface of the tooth.
    A. full-cast crown
    B. partial crown
    C. three-quarter crown
    D. onlay

4. Which cast restoration covers the area between the cusps in the middle of the tooth, the proximal surfaces that are involved, and the cusp ridges? _____
    A. Full-cast crown
    B. Partial crown
    C. Three-quarter crown
    D. Onlay

5. Which cast restoration covers three or more, but not all, surfaces of the tooth? _____
    A. Full-cast crown
    B. Partial crown
    C. Three-quarter crown
    D. Onlay

6. Which restoration replaces the missing tooth structure of a mesio-occlusal surface? _____
    A. Onlay
    B. Inlay
    C. Three-quarter crown
    D. Partial crown

7. The Maryland bridge is used to replace _____ tooth (teeth).
    A. one   C. three
    B. two   D. four

8. _____ are thin layers of tooth-colored material that cover much of the facial surface.
    A. Porcelain-fused-to-metal crowns
    B. Implant retainer prostheses
    C. Core buildups
    D. Veneers

9. Dental casting alloy uses a combination of metals such as _____
    A. silane.   C. platinum.
    B. polysiloxane.   D. polyether.

10. _____ is treatment performed for vital teeth that have very little crown structure and is made of amalgam, composite, or a silver alloy/glass ionomer combination.
    A. Veneer
    B. Core buildup
    C. Retention pin
    D. Post-retained core

11. The dentist performs an examination to determine which patients are candidates for a fixed prosthesis. Which of the following methods are part of the examination? _____
    1. Exam of intra- and extraoral tissues
    2. Number of inlays
    3. Radiographs
    4. Retention pins
    5. Diagnostic casts made
    6. Implant retainer prosthesis

    A. 1, 4, 6
    B. 1, 3, 5
    C. 2, 3, 6
    D. 2, 4, 5

12. A bridge is a restoration that spans the space of a missing tooth or teeth. The teeth adjacent to the missing tooth are called _____
    A. pontics.   B. abutments.

13. Each unit of a bridge represents a tooth. The missing tooth is replaced by a(n) _____
    A. pontic.   B. abutment.

SKILL COMPETENCY ASSESSMENT

24-1 Porcelain Veneers

Student's Name _____ Date _____

Instructor's Name _____

SKILL The technique for the porcelain veneer is sensitive to shade selection and gingival margin adaption if the veneer is to look natural and adapt well. Porcelain veneers are similar to indirect resin veneers in that they require two appointments and are fabricated in the dental laboratory. Routine steps should be followed for all treatment areas to maintain absolute clinical asepsis. The dental assistant must be prepared and thinking ahead to anticipate the dentist's needs.

PERFORMANCE OBJECTIVE The student will follow a routine procedure that meets the regulations and the protocol set forth by the dentist and regulatory agencies, keeping in mind that assistants' duties vary from state to state. The procedure is completed in two appointments. During the first appointment, the tooth is prepared and impressions are taken; the second appointment is the seating of the porcelain veneer. In between the two appointments, the impressions are sent to a dental laboratory where the porcelain veneer is fabricated. The assistant may be evaluated by performance, statement, and/or combined responses and action.

	Self Evaluation	Student Evaluation	Possible Points	Instructor Evaluation	Comments
Equipment and Supplies					
1. Basic setup: mouth mirror, explorer, and cotton pliers			3		
2. Cotton rolls, 2 x 2 gauze			2		
3. HVE tip, air-water syringe tip			3		
4. Anesthetic setup			3		
5. High-speed handpiece and assorted burs			3		
6. Shade guide			3		
7. Spoon excavator			3		
8. Low-speed handpiece with prophy angle, rubber cup, and pumice			3		
9. Retraction cord and placement instrument			3		
10. Bite registration materials			3		
11. Alginate impression materials for model of opposing arch			3		
12. Final impression materials (polysiloxane or polyether)			3		
13. Temporary veneer (optional)			2		
14. Laboratory prescription form			2		
Preparation Appointment (First Appointment)					
Competency Steps					
1. Bite registration taken.			2		
2. Opposing arch impression taken.			3		
3. Teeth cleaned with rubber cup and pumice (remove extrinsic stains).			3		

24-1 continued

	Self Evaluation	Student Evaluation	Possible Points	Instructor Evaluation	Comments
4. Shade selection by dentist (how light patient wants veneers and how light finished shade will be).			3		
5. Teeth prepared according to design of veneer (incisal edge and cervical margin carefully prepared so finished veneer will be even with gingival crest or just slightly subgingival).			3		
6. Retraction cord placed (achieve hemostasis and visualization of margins).			3		
7. Final impression is taken with a dimensionally stable material (polysiloxane or polyether).			3		
8. Temporary veneers are placed if necessary.			3		
9. The retraction cord is removed after temporary veneers are placed.			3		
10. Inform patient that the gums will be tender for several days from the retraction cord placement.			2		
11. Patient is dismissed.			2		
Laboratory Fabrication					
1. Impressions sent to dental laboratory with a laboratory prescription.			3		
2. Laboratory will follow dentist's prescription on length of veneer, shade, thickness, and texture (color photos of patient are helpful in designing and shading process).			3		
3. The laboratory fabricates the veneers and returns them to office.			3		
Cementation Appointment (Second Appointment)					
Equipment and Supplies					
1. Basic setup: mouth mirror, explorer, and cotton pliers			3		
2. Cotton rolls, 2 x 2 gauze, cheek and lip retractors			3		
3. Saliva ejector, HVE tip, air-water syringe tip			3		
4. Porcelain veneers from the laboratory			3		
5. Low-speed handpiece with prophy angle, rubber cup, and pumice			3		
6. Silane coupling agent and small applicator (brush)			3		
7. Retraction cord and placement instrument			3		
8. Chlorhexidine soap			2		
9. Plastic or ultrathin metal strips			2		
10. Etchant and applicator			3		

24-1 continued

	Self Evaluation	Student Evaluation	Possible Points	Instructor Evaluation	Comments
11. Bonding agent and curing light			3		
Competency Steps					
1. Appointment scheduling (coordinated as close as possible to first appointment and laboratory scheduled so turnaround time minimal).			3		
2. Preliminary cleaning of teeth with pumice (remove plaque and stains).			3		
3. Veneers are tried on tooth and adjustments are made with finishing diamonds (veneers are fragile, handle with care).			3		
4. Inside of veneer is cleaned and dried thoroughly (acid etch is used to clean and decontaminate inside of veneer).			3		
5. Apply thin layer of silane coupling agent (this material allows bonding to porcelain).			3		
6. Place light-cured bonding agent in veneers (make sure no air bubbles).			3		
7. Material fills the veneer and is evenly spread around.			3		
8. Veneers are placed in a light-protected area or box until teeth are prepared.			3		
9. Prepare teeth for bonding: A. Place retraction cord on facial surface B. Clean facial surface with chlorhexidine soap C. Prophy cup or brush			3 3 3		
10. Isolate teeth being bonded: A. Cotton rolls B. Cheek and lip retractors C. Saliva ejector D. Plastic or ultrathin metal strips			2 2 2 2		
11. Etch teeth being bonded (follow directions of specific adhesive system).			3		
12. Apply adhesive to teeth being bonded.			3		
13. Each veneer is seated in the correct position.			3		
14. In some cases, veneer is spot cured and excess cement removed.			3		
15. Light cure each veneer in place.			3		
16. Excess cement is removed with scalpel.			3		
17. Margins are contoured and refined with finishing diamonds or burs.			3		

24-1 continued

	Self Evaluation	Student Evaluation	Possible Points	Instructor Evaluation	Comments
18. Veneers are polished with rubber wheels, cups, and polishing paste.			3		

TOTAL POINTS POSSIBLE   174

TOTAL POINTS POSSIBLE—2nd Attempt   172

TOTAL POINTS EARNED   _____

Points assigned reflect importance of step to meeting objective: Important = 1; Essential = 2; Critical = 3. Students will lose 2 points for repeated attempts. Failure results if any of the critical steps are omitted or performed incorrectly. If using a 100-point scale, determine score by dividing points earned by total points possible and multiplying the results by 100.

SCORE: _____

SKILL COMPETENCY ASSESSMENT

24-2 Preparation for a Porcelain-Fused-to-Metal Crown

Student's Name _____ Date _____

Instructor's Name _____

SKILL   The dental assistant assists the dentist in all aspects of the procedure from selecting the shade of the tooth to general chairside assisting. The dental assistant is responsible for preparation of equipment and supplies needed for both appointments. Each tray setup is arranged according to sequence of the procedure, with auxiliary instruments and materials close at hand. The procedure includes many different types of dental materials that the dental assistant will prepare and/or utilize throughout the procedure. The assistant coordinates the patient's appointments and the laboratory schedule. In some offices, the assistant may perform some laboratory functions. In some states with advanced functions, the qualified assistant can perform procedures such as place retraction cord, place and remove temporaries, take preliminary impressions, and remove excess cement.

PERFORMANCE OBJECTIVE   The student will follow a routine procedure that meets the regulations and the protocol set forth by the dentist and regulatory agencies, keeping in mind that assistants' duties vary from state to state. The procedure is performed by the dentist and dental assistant. This process involves two appointments like the porcelain veneer procedure. The following sequence of procedures for a patient needing a porcelain-to-metal crown includes the steps in the preparation appointment, including retention procedures, and the steps in the cementation appointment. Each step is explained and the dental assistant's responsibilities are described. The patient is seated and prepared for the procedure. The assistant may be evaluated by performance, statement, and/or combined responses and action.

	Self Evaluation	Student Evaluation	Possible Points	Instructor Evaluation	Comments
Equipment and Supplies					
1. Basic setup: mouth mirror, explorer, and cotton pliers			3		
2. Cotton rolls, gauze, dental floss, articulating paper, and forceps			3		
3. HVE tip, saliva ejector, and three-way syringe tip			3		
4. Anesthetic setup			3		
5. Dental dam setup			3		
6. High-speed handpiece with selection of diamonds, discs, and burs			3		
7. Irreversible hydrocolloid (alginate) impression materials			3		
8. Spoon excavator, scaler, plastic filling instrument, and cement spatula			3		
9. Tooth shade guide (optional)			2		
10. Retention materials depending on amount of tooth structure retained—core buildup materials and postretention pins (optional)			3		
11. Gingival retraction cord and placement instrument			3		
12. Final impression material and tray (stock or custom tray)			3		
13. Bite registration materials			3		
14. Crown and collar scissors			3		

24-2 continued

	Self Evaluation	Student Evaluation	Possible Points	Instructor Evaluation	Comments
15. Provisional (temporary) coverage materials			3		
16. Low-speed handpiece with burs, discs, and stones			3		
17. Laboratory prescription and container for impressions (off-tray item)			3		
Competency Steps					
1. Local anesthetic administered					
A. Assistant prepares syringe			3		
B. Transfers syringe to dentist			3		
C. Assistant observes patient			3		
2. Alginate impressions for types of temporaries and model of opposing arch:					
A. Assistant selects trays			3		
B. Mixes the irreversible hydrocolloid			3		
C. Takes impression			3		
D. Impressions properly stored and/or poured in plaster or stone			3		
3. Tooth shade guide selection:					
A. Assistant prepares shade guide			2		
B. Assists in selection of shade			2		
C. Records shade selection			3		
4. Crown preparation with high-speed handpiece and various diamond and burs.			3		
5. Margins of preparation finished:					
A. Chamfer or shoulder preparation			3		
B. Assistant prepares and passes the high-speed handpiece			3		
C. Assistant evacuates and maintains operating field with air water syringe			3		
D. Assistant retracts and exchanges instruments such as spoon excavator			3		
6. Retraction cord placement:					
A. Assistant passes a piece of retraction cord in cotton pliers to the dentist			3		
B. Passes the appropriate cord condensing instrument			3		
7. Retraction cord remains in place for five minutes.			3		
8. The dentist selects the tray and impression material to be used.			3		
9. Final impression:					
A. Cotton pliers are passed to remove the retraction cord			3		
B. Syringe material is passed			3		
C. Cotton pliers and cord are received			3		
D. Dentist will seat tray			3		

24-2 continued

	Self Evaluation	Student Evaluation	Possible Points	Instructor Evaluation	Comments
E. Assistant moves light from patient's face and cleans up impression materials			2		
F. Impression materials are rinsed, disinfected, and placed in a plastic laboratory container			3		
10. Bite registration:					
A. Assistant prepares bite registration materials			2		
B. Passes bite registration to dentist (in some states, the dental assistant can legally take the bite impression)			2		
C. After the bite registration is taken, assistant rinses patient's mouth			2		
D. Materials are rinsed, disinfected, and placed in a plastic laboratory container			3		
11. Provisional restoration (temporary):					
A. Purpose			3		
B. Function			3		
C. Esthetic capabilities			3		
D. Length of wear			3		
12. Temporary types:					
A. Crown forms (identification)			3		
B. Custom made (identification)			3		
13. Dentist or assistant will make the temporary restoration depending on the expanded functions laws:					
A. Prepare materials and trays as dictated by technique			3		
B. Equipment and supplies ready:					
1. Crown and bridge scissors			3		
2. Crimping and contour pliers			3		
3. Burs, discs, and stones to contour and finish			3		
C. Assistant passes and receives instruments			3		
D. Keeps area rinsed and dried			3		
E. Assistant mixes the temporary cement			3		
F. Places temporary cement in crown					
G. Passes bite stick for patient to bite on			2		
H. Passes 2 x 2 gauze sponge to wipe off any excess			2		
14. Once cement is dried, bite stick removed.			2		
15. Scaler is used to remove excess dry cement.			3		
16. Dental floss passed to check the interproximal contacts.			3		
17. Assistant holds articulating paper in articulating forceps for patient to bite on to test bite.			2		
18. If adjustments are needed, assistant passes low-speed handpiece with finishing bur.			3		

24-2 continued

	Self Evaluation	Student Evaluation	Possible Points	Instructor Evaluation	Comments
19. Patient's mouth is rinsed and evacuated before the patient is dismissed.			3		
20. After patient is dismissed, patient's impressions, models, and laboratory prescription are ready for the laboratory pickup.			3		
21. Laboratory prescription to include:					
A. Patient's name			3		
B. Description of the prosthesis			3		
C. Types of materials dentist wants prosthesis to be constructed from			3		
D. Shade or shading desired			3		
E. Dentist's name, license number, address, telephone number, fax number, and signature			3		
F. Completion date, when the case will be back in the dental office			3		

TOTAL POINTS POSSIBLE   211

TOTAL POINTS POSSIBLE—2nd Attempt   209

TOTAL POINTS EARNED   _____

Points assigned reflect importance of step to meeting objective: Important = 1; Essential = 2; Critical = 3. Students will lose 2 points for repeated attempts. Failure results if any of the critical steps are omitted or performed incorrectly. If using a 100-point scale, determine score by dividing points earned by total points possible and multiplying the results by 100.

SCORE: _____

SKILL COMPETENCY ASSESSMENT

24-3 Cementation of Porcelain-Fused-to-Metal Crown

Student's Name _____ Date _____

Instructor's Name _____

SKILL   The dental assistant is responsible for preparation of equipment and supplies needed for the appointment. The procedure includes removal of the temporary restoration and cementation of the permanent prosthesis.

PERFORMANCE OBJECTIVE   The student will follow a routine procedure that meets the regulations and the protocol set forth by the dentist and regulatory agencies, keeping in mind that assistants' duties vary from state to state. The temporary is removed and the permanent prosthesis is evaluated and the final cementation is completed. The assistant may be evaluated by performance, statement, and/or combined responses and action.

	Self Evaluation	Student Evaluation	Possible Points	Instructor Evaluation	Comments
Equipment and Supplies					
1. Basic setup: mouth mirror, explorer, and cotton pliers			3		
2. Cotton rolls, gauze, dental floss, articulating paper, and forceps			3		
3. HVE tip, saliva ejector, and air-water syringe tip			3		
4. Low-speed handpiece with finishing burs, discs, and stones			3		
5. Anesthetic setup			3		
6. Spoon excavator and scaler			3		
7. Plastic filling instrument (PFI)			3		
8. Orangewood bite stick (crown remover, crown seater, and mallet are optional)			3		
9. Final cementation materials (glass ionomer cement, polycarboxylate cement, resin cements, or zinc phosphate cement)			2		
10. Porcelain-fused-to-metal crown from laboratory			3		
Competency Steps					
1. Day before appointment, make sure laboratory has completed crown and it is at office.			3		
2. Assistant prepares topical and local anesthetic.			3		
3. Transfers syringe to dentist.			3		
4. Observes patient.			3		
5. Assistant rinses and evacuates the mouth.			3		
6. Provisional coverage is removed with a crown remover, scaler, and other instruments of choice (ones that fit under the margin of temporary).			3		
7. Assistant either assists during removal of temporary and excess cement removal by transferring instruments and keeping area clean and free of debris			3		

24-3 continued

	Self Evaluation	Student Evaluation	Possible Points	Instructor Evaluation	Comments
or as part of expanded functions					
8. Assistant removes temporary.			3		
9. Assistant removes excess cement.			3		
10. Assistant rinses and dries the area and readies crown.			3		
11. Casting try-in:					
A. Assistant transfers instruments			3		
B. Transfers dental floss			2		
C. Transfers articulating paper and forceps			2		
D. Assistant keeps area dry			3		
E. Passes low-speed handpiece with finishing burs, discs, and stones			3		
F. If casting has to be returned to laboratory, the assistant will disinfect crown and prepare it to return to laboratory			3		
12. Prior to cementation, the area is isolated with cotton rolls and protective liners and/or a cavity varnish is placed.			3		
13. Permanent cement materials are ready and will be mixed according to manufacturer's directions.			3		
14. Assistant mixes permanent cement when dentist is ready.			3		
15. Assistant places some cement in crown and passes to dentist.			3		
16. Assistant passes plastic filling instrument to dentist to place cement on preparation.			3		
17. Assistant receives PFI and passes crown.			3		
18. Assistant passes bite stick for patient to bite.			2		
19. After cement has hardened, excess cement is removed with a scaler or an explorer.			3		
20. Patient's mouth is rinsed and evacuated.			2		
21. Dental floss is used to remove excess cement interproximally.			3		
22. Patient is given instructions on brushing and flossing.			3		
23. Assistant documents procedure, and patient is dismissed.			3		

TOTAL POINTS POSSIBLE   109

TOTAL POINTS POSSIBLE—2nd Attempt   107

TOTAL POINTS EARNED   _____

Points assigned reflect importance of step to meeting objective: Important = 1; Essential = 2; Critical = 3. Students will lose 2 points for repeated attempts. Failure results if any of the critical steps are omitted or performed incorrectly. If using a 100-point scale, determine score by dividing points earned by total points possible and multiplying the results by 100.

SCORE: _____

Removable Prosthodontics

The student should strive to meet the following objectives and demonstrate an understanding of the facts and principles presented in this chapter:

1. Define removable prostheses and list the reasons for using them.
2. Describe the patient considerations related to removable prosthetic treatment.
3. Explain the dental assistant's role in removable prosthetic treatment.
4. Outline the steps of the diagnostic appointment and list the materials needed.
5. Describe the consultation appointment and the materials required for the case presentation.
6. Describe the advantages and disadvantages of the partial denture, the components, and the appointment schedule.
7. Describe the complete denture, the patient considerations, and the appointment schedule.
8. Explain the types and steps of denture reline procedures.
9. Describe the procedure for a denture repair.
10. List the steps to polish a removable prosthetic appliance.
11. Explain the overdenture and the advantages and disadvantages related to it.

SUMMARY

Removable prosthodontics, like fixed prosthodontics, refers to the replacement of missing teeth and tissues with artificial structures, or prostheses. With removable prosthodontics, however, the prosthesis can be removed from the mouth by the patient. Most patients prefer to have fixed prostheses, but in some cases it may not be the treatment of choice due to existing conditions.

The dental assistant's main functions are to prepare materials, record measurements and details for the fabrication of the denture, provide patient education and support, and perform some laboratory procedures. The procedures in removable prosthodontics do not require many instrument exchanges, and the assistant does not continually maintain the oral cavity throughout the appointment with the air-water syringe and the HVE. The steps in removable prosthodontics involve as many extraoral as intraoral procedures. The dental assistant has all of the items prepared so that the dentist can explain the diagnosis, the proposed treatment plan, and the prognosis to the patient.

KEY TERMS

abutment	connectors	partial dentures
anatomical	denture base	prostheses
baseplate	framework	relined
bite rim	muscle trimming	rests
border molding	non-anatomical	retainer
centric occlusion	overdenture	vertical dimension

EXERCISES AND ACTIVITIES

1. To be successful with a removable prosthetic appliance, a patient should _____
   A. have a positive attitude.
   B. be cooperative.
   C. be able to maintain good oral hygiene.
   D. be mentally prepared.
   E. All of the above

2. Which of the following is a benefit of a removable partial appliance? _____
   A. If teeth are lost, they can be added to partial
   B. No oral hygiene maintenance
   C. No support to teeth standing alone
   D. Frequent adjustment

3. Before choosing a partial denture, the dentist must determine which of the following? _____
   A. Whether there is adequate root structure of the remaining teeth
   B. Whether the patient can maintain good oral health
   C. Whether the alveolar bone structure is adequate
   D. All of the above

4. The _____ are the part of the removable partial denture that are positioned on the occlusal, incisal or cingulum surfaces.
   A. connectors   C. retainers
   B. stress-breakers   D. rests

5. Which of the following is not a portion of the metal framework skeleton on a removable partial? _____
   A. Rests   C. Connectors
   B. Acrylic   D. Retainers

6. What portion of the metal framework holds the working parts in the proper position? _____
   A. Rests   C. Connectors
   B. Stress-breaker D. Clasps

7. What portion of the partial is most often made of acrylic resin and holds the denture teeth in the dental base? _____
   A. Stress-breaker C. Retainer
   B. Connector   D. Saddle

8. The _____ where the metal framework of the partial rests must be prepared before the final impressions are taken.
   A. saddle
   B. border molding
   C. abutment teeth
   D. centric occlusion

9. The dental laboratory _____ the appliance on models to simulate how it will occlude and mesh in various jaw positions.
   A. relines   C. trims
   B. articulates   D. cleans

10. What is a characteristic of anatomical posterior denture teeth? _____
    A. Resemble natural teeth with cusps
    B. No detailed anatomy on occlusal
    C. Concave
    D. Flat

11. The patient moves mouth, lips, cheeks, and tongue to establish accurate length for periphery and adjacent tissues to be included in the final impression. This is called _____
    A. bite rim.
    B. centric occlusion.
    C. muscle trimming.
    D. vertical dimension.

12. What is the preformed, semi-rigid, acrylic resin material that temporarily represents the denture base? _____
    A. Baselate
    B. Bite rim
    C. Vertical dimension
    D. Centric occlusion

13. In the natural dentition, the length of the crowns of the teeth determines the distance between the upper and lower jaws. This distance is called the _____
    A. centric occlusion.
    B. vertical dimension.
    C. border molding.
    D. denture base.

14. What is determined when the jaws are closed in a position that produces maximum contact between the occluding surfaces of the maxillary and mandibular arch? _____

    A. Centric occlusion
    B. Vertical dimension
    C. Border molding
    D. Denture base

15. When pressure from a complete or partial denture causes the supporting tissues to shrink and change in size, the procedure to improve the fit of the denture and comfort of the patient is called _____

    A. overdenture.
    B. try-in.
    C. relining.
    D. muscle trim.

16. Which of the following items is required for a consultation appointment? _____

    1. Baseplate
    2. Try-in
    3. Study models of patient's mouth
    4. Radiographs mounted on viewbox
    5. Contour pliers
    6. Proposed treatment plan

    A. 1, 2, 5
    B. 3, 4, 6
    C. 2, 3, 5
    D. 1, 3, 4

SKILL COMPETENCY ASSESSMENT

25-1 Final Impression Appointment *(corresponds to textbook Procedure 25-4)*

Student's Name _____ Date _____

Instructor's Name _____

SKILL   The dental assistant is responsible for preparation of equipment and supplies needed for the appointment. Between the consultation and the final impressions appointment, the alginate impressions are poured in plaster or stone. On these models, custom acrylic trays are constructed.

PERFORMANCE OBJECTIVE   The student will follow a routine procedure that meets the regulations and the protocol set forth by the dentist and regulatory agencies, keeping in mind that assistants' duties vary from state to state. The assistant may be evaluated by performance, statement, and/or combined responses and action. The procedure is performed by the dentist. Materials are prepared and passed to the dentist by the dental assistant.

	Self Evaluation	Student Evaluation	Possible Points	Instructor Evaluation	Comments
Equipment and Supplies					
1. Basic setup: mouth mirror, explorer, and cotton pliers			3		
2. HVE tip, air-water syringe tip			3		
3. Cotton rolls and gauze			3		
4. Mouthwash for patient to rinse prior to impressions being taken			3		
5. Custom tray			3		
6. Compound wax and Bunsen burner for border molding the rims of the trays			3		
7. Laboratory knife to trim border molding			2		
8. Impression materials—spatulas and mixing pads or dispensing gun and tips			3		
9. Laboratory prescription form			2		
10. Disinfectant and container for impressions and bite registration			3		
Competency Steps					
1. Custom tray inserted into patient's mouth (assistant may pass tray to dentist) and evaluated for fit.			3		
2. Border molding or muscle trimming takes place (impression compound heated, placed along borders of custom tray, tray is then cooled, placed in patient's mouth, while tray is in patient's mouth—lips, cheeks, and tongue are moved to establish accurate length of periphery and adjacent tissue to be included in final impression).			3		

25-1 continued *(corresponds to textbook Procedure 25-4)*

	Self Evaluation	Student Evaluation	Possible Points	Instructor Evaluation	Comments
3. Assistant prepares final impression material and places into tray.			3		
Maxillary impression evaluation (include tuberosities, frenum attachments, other landmarks of the arch)			3		
Mandibular impression evaluation (include retromolar pads, oblique ridge, mylohyoid ridge, and frenum attachments)			3		
4. Tray is removed once material has set.			3		
5. Assistant rinses patient's mouth thoroughly.			3		
6. Impression procedure is repeated for opposing arch if full denture is being fabricated for both arches.			3		
7. Impressions are disinfected and prepared for the laboratory.			3		
8. The prescription form is prepared and sent to the laboratory.			2		
9. Patient is dismissed.			2		

TOTAL POINTS POSSIBLE   59

TOTAL POINTS POSSIBLE—2nd Attempt   57

TOTAL POINTS EARNED   _____

Points assigned reflect importance of step to meeting objective: Important = 1; Essential = 2; Critical = 3. Students will lose 2 points for repeated attempts. Failure results if any of the critical steps are omitted or performed incorrectly. If using a 100-point scale, determine score by dividing points earned by total points possible and multiplying the results by 100.

SCORE: _____

SKILL COMPETENCY ASSESSMENT

25-2 Jaw Relationship Appointment *(corresponds to textbook Procedure 25-5)*

Student's Name _____ Date _____

Instructor's Name _____

SKILL The dental assistant is responsible for preparation of equipment and supplies needed for the appointment. Between the final impressions appointment and the measurement appointment, the dental laboratory pours the master cast in stone from the final impressions. The master cast will be used to construct the baseplate. Attached to the baseplate will be the bite rim. Once the baseplate and bite rims are constructed, they are sent to the dental office ready for this appointment.

PERFORMANCE OBJECTIVE The student will follow a routine procedure that meets the regulations and the protocol set forth by the dentist and regulatory agencies, keeping in mind that assistants' duties vary from state to state. The assistant may be evaluated by performance, statement and/or combined responses and action. During this appointment, measurements, shape, and shade of the denture are determined. The dental assistant prepares equipment and materials and assists the dentist throughout the procedure.

	Self Evaluation	Student Evaluation	Possible Points	Instructor Evaluation	Comments
Equipment and Supplies					
1. Basic setup: mouth mirror, explorer, and cotton pliers			3		
2. HVE tip, air-water syringe tip			3		
3. Hand mirror			2		
4. Laboratory knife, #7 wax spatula, Bunsen burner			3		
5. Shade guide			3		
6. Millimeter ruler and boley gauge			3		
7. Baseplates and bite rims			3		
8. Face bow			3		
9. Photographs of the patient, showing the shape and shade of the teeth			3		
10. Laboratory prescription form			2		
11. Disinfectant			3		
Competency Steps					
1. Baseplates and bite rims inserted into patient's mouth (assistant may pass to dentist). Dentist determines and marks midline of maxillary and mandibular arches.			3		
2. Vertical dimension is determined			3		
A. Bite rims adjusted with laboratory knife (length of crowns of teeth/distance between upper and lower jaws)			3		
B. Patient natural lip line determined			3		
C. Correct amount of tooth and gingiva visible when talking and smiling and the lips are in resting position			3		
D. Cuspid lines determined at corners of mouth			3		

25-2 continued *(corresponds to textbook Procedure 25-5)*

	Self Evaluation	Student Evaluation	Possible Points	Instructor Evaluation	Comments
3. Centric occlusion is determined			3		
A. Jaw relationship evaluated how mandible relates to maxilla			3		
B. Patient moves mandible to retrusion (back)			3		
C. Patient moves mandible to lateral movement (right to left/side to side)			3		
D. Once determined information is correct, casts will articulate to duplicate normal motions of patient			3		
E. Laboratory technician constructs complete denture in wax and with artificial teeth from these records			3		
4. Denture teeth selected			3		
A. Arrangement of teeth discussed with patient			3		
B. Proper shade and use of natural light			3		
C. Shade compared with patient's complexion			3		
D. Shade compared with remaining teeth			3		
E. Shade compared with photographs			3		
F. Age of patient indicates shade range			3		
G. Teeth staining sometimes darker with age			3		
H. Shape mold of teeth by face of patient			3		
5. Developing clear communication with patient is important for a successful outcome			3		
A. Natural appearance of teeth			3		
B. Duplicate arrangement of existing teeth (spacing, overlapping, etc.)			3		
C. Correct alignment of natural teeth with new denture			3		
D. Patient clear on expected outcome			3		
6. Patient is dismissed.			2		

TOTAL POINTS POSSIBLE   111

TOTAL POINTS POSSIBLE—2nd Attempt   109

TOTAL POINTS EARNED   _____

Points assigned reflect importance of step to meeting objective: Important = 1; Essential = 2; Critical = 3. Students will lose 2 points for repeated attempts. Failure results if any of the critical steps are omitted or performed incorrectly. If using a 100-point scale, determine score by dividing points earned by total points possible and multiplying the results by 100.

SCORE: _____

SKILL COMPETENCY ASSESSMENT

25-3 The Try-In Appointment (corresponds to textbook Procedure 25-6)

Student's Name _____ Date _____

Instructor's Name _____

SKILL   The dental assistant is responsible for preparation of equipment and supplies needed for the appointment. Between appointments, the laboratory will prepare a "try-in" denture. Denture teeth are mounted in the wax bite rim. They are positioned according to the dentist's directions, but the position can be altered at the try-in appointment.

PERFORMANCE OBJECTIVE   The student will follow a routine procedure that meets the regulations and the protocol set forth by the dentist and regulatory agencies, keeping in mind that assistants' duties vary from state to state. The assistant may be evaluated by performance, statement, and/or combined responses and action. The procedure is performed by the dentist. The dental assistant prepares the patient, the instruments, and materials and coordinates with the dental laboratory.

	Self Evaluation	Student Evaluation	Possible Points	Instructor Evaluation	Comments
Equipment and Supplies					
1. Basic setup: mouth mirror, explorer, and cotton pliers			3		
2. HVE tip, air-water syringe tip			3		
3. Hand mirror			2		
4. Laboratory knife, #7 wax spatula, Bunsen burner			3		
5. Shade guide			3		
6. Millimeter ruler and boley gauge			3		
7. Baseplates and bite rims			3		
8. Face bow			3		
9. Photographs of the patient, showing the shape and shade of the teeth			3		
10. Laboratory prescription form			2		
11. Disinfectant			3		
Competency Steps					
1. "Try-in" denture is disinfected before being placed in patient's mouth.			3		
2. Patient is seated.			2		
3. Denture inserted into patient's mouth.			3		
4. Time will be spent talking to allow patient to adjust to denture.			3		
5. Denture is evaluated for esthetics, retention, and comfort.			3		
6. Occlusion is checked with articulating paper (assistant will transfer as needed).			3		
7. Dentist can adjust the position of the teeth because they are still in wax.			3		

25-3 continued *(corresponds to textbook Procedure 25-6)*

	Self Evaluation	Student Evaluation	Possible Points	Instructor Evaluation	Comments
8. The shade can be changed by dental laboratory technician in the dental laboratory.			3		
9. Once dentist and patient are satisfied with denture, the denture will be disinfected and placed back onto the articulator.			3		
10. The denture is returned to the laboratory.			2		
11. PATIENT IS DISMISSED.			2		

TOTAL POINTS POSSIBLE   61

TOTAL POINTS POSSIBLE—2nd Attempt   59

TOTAL POINTS EARNED   _____

Points assigned reflect importance of step to meeting objective: Important = 1; Essential = 2; Critical = 3. Students will lose 2 points for repeated attempts. Failure results if any of the critical steps are omitted or performed incorrectly. If using a 100-point scale, determine score by dividing points earned by total points possible and multiplying the results by 100.

SCORE: _____

SKILL COMPETENCY ASSESSMENT

25-4 Denture Relining *(corresponds to textbook Procedure 25-8)*

Student's Name _____ Date _____

Instructor's Name _____

SKILL   The dental assistant is responsible for preparation of equipment and supplies needed for the appointment. The denture relining adds a new layer of acrylic to the inside of the denture. This procedure can be done in the dental office or at the dental laboratory. Both methods are a part of this assessment.

PERFORMANCE OBJECTIVE   The student will follow a routine procedure that meets the regulations and the protocol set forth by the dentist and regulatory agencies, keeping in mind that assistants' duties vary from state to state. The assistant may be evaluated by performance, statement, and/or combined responses and action. The dental assistant prepares the patient and the materials.

	Self Evaluation	Student Evaluation	Possible Points	Instructor Evaluation	Comments
Equipment and Supplies					
1. Basic setup: mouth mirror, explorer, and cotton pliers			3		
2. Low-speed handpiece with acrylic burs			3		
3. Chairside reline materials			3		
4. Mouth rinse			2		
Chairside Relining Competency Steps					
1. Prepare denture, place in ultrasonic unit for a few minutes to be cleaned.			3		
2. Dentist uses acrylic burs to roughen tissue side of denture.			3		
3. Either hard or semi-soft reline materials available for doctor to choose.			3		
4. Material mixed to manufacturer's direction.			3		
5. Place material in clean denture, covering entire tissue surface (materials have low thermal reaction and can cure directly in patient's mouth).			3		
6. Patient rinses with mouthwash to clean saliva and debris from tissues.			3		
7. Denture is inserted in patient's mouth and patient is asked to bite until initial set stage (patient will be told there is sometimes a slight burning sensation from the acrylic material during setting time).			3		
8. Denture is removed to complete setting process.			3		
9. Dentist will trim away excess material.			3		
10. After adjustments, the denture is polished in the laboratory before being returned to patient.			3		
11. If adjustments are made, the denture will need to be disinfected before replacing it in patient's mouth.			3		

25-4 continued *(corresponds to textbook Procedure 25-8)*

	Self Evaluation	Student Evaluation	Possible Points	Instructor Evaluation	Comments

Dental Laboratory Relining

PERFORMANCE OBJECTIVE   The patient's denture is prepared in the same manner as for the chairside relining procedure. The following are the impression and laboratory steps. The tray setup is the same as that in the chairside relining, except for the type of materials used.

Competency Steps

	Self Evaluation	Student Evaluation	Possible Points	Instructor Evaluation	Comments
1. Denture or partial is used for the impression materials.			3		
2. Impression materials available include polysulfides, polyethers, and silicone (assistant will need to be prepared to mix any of these).			3		
3. Impression material of choice mixed according to manufacturer's direction.			3		
4. Material placed in tray. Material should cover entire tissue surface evenly and without excess.			3		
5. Denture is inserted into patient's mouth and positioned firmly (patient to occlude and hold until material is set).			3		
6. After material is set, denture is removed from patient's mouth.			2		
7. Denture is disinfected and prepared to be sent to dental laboratory.			3		
8. Laboratory prescription is completed.			3		
9. Patient is dismissed.			2		
10. Dental laboratory will process impression (acrylic resin base fused to denture).			2		
11. Patient returns to dental office when laboratory completes process of denture reline (turn-around time varies from hours to days).			2		
12. When patient returns to the dental office, denture is seated.			3		
13. Denture adjustments are made as needed.			3		
14. After adjustments, the denture is polished in the laboratory before returning to patient.			3		
15. If adjustments are made, the denture will need to be disinfected before replacing it in patient's mouth.			3		
16. Patient is dismissed.			2		

TOTAL POINTS POSSIBLE			87		
TOTAL POINTS POSSIBLE—2nd Attempt			85		
TOTAL POINTS EARNED			_____		

Points assigned reflect importance of step to meeting objective: Important = 1; Essential = 2; Critical = 3. Students will lose 2 points for repeated attempts. Failure results if any of the critical steps are omitted or performed incorrectly. If using a 100-point scale, determine score by dividing points earned by total points possible and multiplying the results by 100.

SCORE: _____

Chairside Restorative Materials

OBJECTIVES

The student should strive to meet the following objectives and demonstrate an understanding of the facts and principles presented in this chapter:

1. Explain the types of dental restorative materials.
2. List the standards and organizations responsible for the standards.
3. Explain the role of the dental assistant.
4. List and explain the properties of dental materials.
5. List the types of materials used to restore cavity preparations.
6. Identify the types of dental cements. Explain their properties, composition, uses, and manipulation.
7. Describe bonding agents and their manipulation.
8. Identify the types of direct restorative materials and where they are used.
9. Describe the steps of cavity preparation.
10. Identify cavity preparation terminology.
11. Explain the properties, composition, and manipulation of dental amalgam.
12. Identify the armamentarium and steps of an amalgam procedure.
13. Explain the composition of composite resins.
14. Explain the properties and manipulation of various cavity classifications.
15. Identify the armamentarium and steps of a composite restoration.
16. Explain the use of glass ionomer resin restorative materials.

SUMMARY

The general chairside assistant prepares and mixes the material, while the dentist places the material in the oral cavity. Some states allow the assistant to also place the material in the oral cavity. Knowledge of the properties of the dental material is necessary for the dental assistant to properly prepare and manipulate the materials. The dental assistant's knowledge of dental materials is beneficial for patient education and protection. Expanded-function dental assistants must understand and be competent in the placement and finishing of the materials.

KEY TERMS

acid etchant	corrosion	luting	smear layer
adhesives	dimensional change	malleability	soluble
alloy	dual-cured materials	mechanical retention	strain
amalgam	ductility	microleakage	stress
base	exothermic	primer	thermal property
bonding agents	flow	polycarboxylate	varnish
calcium hydroxide	galvanism	resin cements	viscosity
cavosurface margin	glass ionomer	sedative or palliative	wettability
composite	light cured	effect	zinc oxide eugenol
compules	liner	self-curing	zinc phosphate

EXERCISES AND ACTIVITIES

1. An example of shearing stress and strain is _____, or grinding of the teeth.
   A. dimensional change
   B. corrosion
   C. tarnish
   D. bruxism

2. Which of the following is not a type of stress and strain? _____
   A. Tensile
   B. Dimensional
   C. Compressive
   D. Shearing

3. The ability of a material to withstand compressive stresses without fracturing is known as _____
   A. malleability.
   B. ductility.
   C. palliative.
   D. viscosity.

4. _____ is the result of chemical or electrochemical attacks of the oral environment on pure metal, causing deep pitting and roughness.
   A. Tarnishing
   B. Corrosion
   C. Shearing
   D. Ductility

5. _____ is the ability to be distorted or deformed by an applied force and then returned to the original shape once the force is removed.
   A. Flow
   B. Retention
   C. Elasticity
   D. Solubility

6. _____, or creep and slump, is a continuing deformation of a solid.
   A. Flow
   B. Elasticity
   C. Solubility
   D. Ductility

7. A dental material can change from a variety of causes. Which of the following is not a cause of dimensional change? _____
   A. Tarnish
   B. Setting process
   C. Exposure to cold
   D. Exposure to heat

8. When saliva and debris from the oral cavity seep between the tooth structure and the restorative materials, this is known as _____
   A. flow.
   B. ductility.
   C. malleability.
   D. microleakage.

9. The ability of material to transmit heat is called _____
   A. dimensional change.
   B. microleakage.
   C. thermal conductivity.
   D. stress and strain.

10. What property may make a dental material useful as a base or liner, where it is not exposed to the oral fluids? _____
    A. Viscosity
    B. Solubility
    C. Wettability
    D. Galvanism

11. In dentistry, materials that are placed directly into the cavity preparation (direct restorative materials) are kept in place by _____
    A. chemical retention.
    B. mechanical retention.
    C. viscosity.
    D. stress and strain.

12. The thicker the material, the less it flows; therefore, it is said to be more _____ than a thin material that flows easily.
    A. viscous
    B. wettable
    C. luting
    D. soluble

13. The ability of a material to flow over a surface is called _____
    A. viscosity.
    B. wettability.
    C. luting.
    D. solubility.

14. Dental cements are mixed to a precise ratio. Zinc phosphate cement has reached the _____ stage when the material will follow the spatula about one inch above the mixing slab.
    A. luting
    B. base
    C. liner
    D. putty

15. What material is placed as a thin layer on the walls and floor of cavity preparation to protect pulp from bacteria and irritants? _____
    A. Base
    B. Liner
    C. Cement
    D. Varnish

16. Bases are applied between the tooth and the restoration to protect the pulp. Which of the following will the base not protect the pulp from? _____
    A. Chemical irritation
    B. Temperature change
    C. Sedation of pulp
    D. Mechanical injury

17. One of the oldest cements, which comes in a powder/liquid form and is a luting and base cement, is called _____
    A. zinc oxide eugenol.
    B. polycarboxylate.
    C. glass ionomer.
    D. zinc phosphate.

18. When zinc phosphate powder and liquid are mixed together, a chemical reaction occurs and heat is released. The reaction is called _____
    A. exothermic.   C. light cure.
    B. viscosity.   D. mechanical.

19. Glass ionomer material has the following properties except _____
    A. mechanically bonds to tooth structure.
    B. chemically bonds to tooth structure.
    C. has non-irritating qualities.
    D. comes with a solvent.

20. Bonding agents bond to all of the following except _____
    A. varnish.   C. dentin.
    B. enamel.   D. porcelain.

21. What cement is said to be "kind" to the pulp and was the first cement that had the ability to chemically bond to the tooth structure? _____
    A. Composite   C. Amalgam
    B. Polycarboxylate   D. Mechanical

22. Adhesion of dental materials to enamel is accomplished by _____
    A. dimensional change.
    B. acid etching.
    C. exothermic reaction.
    D. mechanical retention.

23. This layer of debris prevents contact between intact dentin and the bonding agent/adhesive and is called _____
    A. a smear layer.
    B. a liner.
    C. microleakage.
    D. a sedative.

24. The angle that is formed by the junction of the wall of the preparation and the untouched surface of the tooth is called the _____
    A. line angle.
    B. axial wall.
    C. cavosurface margin.
    D. pulpal floor.

25. Trituration is the _____ means of combining the dental alloy and mercury.
    A. mechanical   C. light cure
    B. chemical   D. self-cure

26. What material dominates the field of esthetic restorations? _____
    A. Glass ionomer
    B. Composite
    C. Bonding agents
    D. Polycarboxylate

27. Materials to prepare the teeth for the actual restoration include which of the following? _____
    1. Amalgam
    2. Bases
    3. Composite
    4. Bonding agents
    5. Microfill composites
    6. Cements

    A. 1, 3, 5
    B. 2, 4, 5
    C. 2, 4, 6
    D. 1, 3, 6

28. The reaction of an object to resist external force is called _____
    A. strain.   B. stress.

29. Which dental cement cures by a chemical reaction between two materials? _____
    A. Self-curing   B. Light curing

30. Which of the cured materials is used with endodontic spots? _____
    A. Self-curing   B. Light curing

SKILL COMPETENCY ASSESSMENT

26-1 Mixing Zinc Phosphate Cement

Student's Name _____ Date _____

Instructor's Name _____

SKILL   The dental assistant is responsible for preparation of equipment and supplies needed for the appointment. Zinc oxide phosphate cement is one of the oldest cements, and although it does have some disadvantages, it is still a reliable choice for a luting and base cement. It comes in a powder/liquid form, and there are several different brands available. One objective in mixing the cement is to dissipate the heat from the exothermic reaction. If the heat is dissipated, the setting reaction is slowed and more powder can be incorporated to make the cement stronger.

PERFORMANCE OBJECTIVE   The student will follow a routine procedure that meets the regulations and the protocol set forth by the dentist and regulatory agencies, keeping in mind that assistants' duties vary from state to state. The assistant may be evaluated by performance, statement, and/or combined responses and action. This procedure is completed by the dental assistant for the dentist. The equipment and materials are prepared, and the material is mixed and passed to the dentist. Sometimes the assistant places the cement in the cast restoration while the dentist places material on the prepared tooth.

	Self Evaluation	Student Evaluation	Possible Points	Instructor Evaluation	Comments
Equipment and Supplies					
1. Zinc phosphate powder and liquid (dispensers, if needed)			3		
2. Cooled glass slab			3		
3. Flexible stainless steel cement spatula			3		
4. 2 x 2 gauze sponge			3		
5. Timer			2		
6. Plastic filling instrument			3		
Competency Steps					
1. Shake powder before removing cap.			3		
2. Place appropriate amount of powder on one end of slab (powder/liquid ratio amount determined by procedure—crown/bridge).			3		
3. Level powder with flat side of spatula blade (layer about 1 mm thick).			3		
4. Divide powder according to manufacturer's directions (divide powder into two equal portions with edge of spatula—continue to divide down to eighths).			3		
5. Gently shake liquid. Dispense liquid onto glass slab; recap to prevent spilling and evaporation (dispense liquid to opposite side of slab—hold vertical to dispense uniform drops).			3		
6. Incorporate one small portion of powder into liquid. Use flat side of spatula blade to wet powder (follow specific manufacturer's directions, about fifteen seconds).			3		
7. Spatulate the powder and liquid over large area of the glass slab (hold spatula blade flat against slab and use wide sweeping motion).			3		

26-1 continued

	Self Evaluation	Student Evaluation	Possible Points	Instructor Evaluation	Comments
8. Add small amounts of powder to liquid and achieve a smooth consistency (incorporate each increment of powder thoroughly before adding more powder—helps to neutralize acid).			3		
9. Mix will appear watery at first. As more powder is incorporated, mix will become creamy (gather all particles of powder and liquid from around edges of mix from time to time).			3		
10. Turn spatula blade on edge and gather mass to check consistency.			3		
11. Continue to add additional increments into mix until desired consistency is reached and within the prescribed time.			3		
12. Gather entire mass into one unit on glass slab.			3		
13. Consistency for luting (cementing) will be creamy (follow spatula for about one inch as lifted off glass slab before breaking into thin thread and flowing back into mass).			3		
14. Consistency of base (putty-like)—can be rolled into ball or cylinder with flat side of spatula.			3		
15. Once cement has been mixed to desired consistency, wipe spatula off with 2 x 2 gauze			2		
16. Hold glass slab under patient's chin and pass plastic filling instrument.			3		
17. Assistant receives plastic filling instrument and wipes it and glass slab off with moistened 2 x 2 gauze.			3		
18. Clean glass slab and spatula (soak in water or solution of bicarbonate of soda to loosen hardened cement and then sterilize/disinfect accordingly).			3		

TOTAL POINTS POSSIBLE   70

TOTAL POINTS POSSIBLE—2nd Attempt   68

TOTAL POINTS EARNED   _____

Points assigned reflect importance of step to meeting objective: Important = 1; Essential = 2; Critical = 3. Students will lose 2 points for repeated attempts. Failure results if any of the critical steps are omitted or performed incorrectly. If using a 100-point scale, determine score by dividing points earned by total points possible and multiplying the results by 100.

SCORE: _____

SKILL COMPETENCY ASSESSMENT

26-2 Mixing Zinc Oxide Eugenol Cement—Powder/Liquid Form

Student's Name _____ Date _____

Instructor's Name _____

SKILL   The dental assistant is responsible for preparation of equipment and supplies needed for appointments. Zinc oxide eugenol, often referred to as ZOE cement, is another cement that has been used for many years. It is noted for its sedative or soothing effect on the dental pulp. The functions of this cement are diverse because of additives that enhance the properties. There are two types. Zinc oxide eugenol comes in several forms including powder/liquid, two-paste systems, capsules, and syringes.

PERFORMANCE OBJECTIVE   The student will follow a routine procedure that meets the regulations and the protocol set forth by the dentist and regulatory agencies, keeping in mind that assistants' duties vary from state to state. The assistant may be evaluated by performance, statement, and/or combined responses and action. This procedure is completed by the dental assistant when the dentist signals. The equipment and materials are prepared, and the material is mixed and passed to the dentist. The assistant follows the manufacturer's directions for specific information on proportions, incorporation technique, and the mixing and setting time.

	Self Evaluation	Student Evaluation	Possible Points	Instructor Evaluation	Comments
Equipment and Supplies					
1. Zinc oxide eugenol cement			3		
2. Dispensers specific to material			2		
3. Paper pad or glass slab			3		
4. Cement spatula			3		
5. Timer			2		
6. Plastic filling instrument			3		
7. 2 x 2 gauze sponges			2		
8. Alcohol or orange solvent			2		
Competency Steps					
1. Fluff powder before removing cap.			3		
2. Place powder on mixing pad (follow manufacturer's directions, and replace cap to avoid spilling and contamination).			3		
3. After swirling, place liquid on paper pad (hold dispensing dropper perpendicular to mixing pad and dispense drops—dispense near powder but not touching).			3		
4. Incorporate powder into liquid in divided increments or all at once (according to manufacturer's directions).			3		
5. Spatulate with flat part of blade, even pressure to "wet" all particles (some cements require firm pressure).			3		
6. Gather up powder and liquid from edges of mix.			3		
7. Gather up entire mass into one unit on slab to test consistency.			3		
8. Consistency for temporary luting will be creamy, like frosting.			3		

26-2 continued

	Self Evaluation	Student Evaluation	Possible Points	Instructor Evaluation	Comments
9. Consistency for insulating base or IRM will be putty-like and can be rolled into a ball or cylinder.			3		
10. Once material has been mixed to desired consistency, wipe spatula with 2 x 2 gauze			2		
11. Hold pad under the patient's chin and pass plastic filling instrument.			3		
12. Assistant receives plastic filling instrument and wipes it off.			3		
13. Top paper pad is removed and folded to prevent accidentally contacting cement.			2		
14. To clean material that has hardened on spatula or glass slab, wipe it with alcohol or orange solvent.			3		

TOTAL POINTS POSSIBLE   60

TOTAL POINTS POSSIBLE—2nd Attempt   58

TOTAL POINTS EARNED   _____

Points assigned reflect importance of step to meeting objective: Important = 1; Essential = 2; Critical = 3. Students will lose 2 points for repeated attempts. Failure results if any of the critical steps are omitted or performed incorrectly. If using a 100-point scale, determine score by dividing points earned by total points possible and multiplying the results by 100.

SCORE: _____

SKILL COMPETENCY ASSESSMENT

26-3 Mixing Polycarboxylate Cement *(corresponds to textbook Procedure 26-4)*

Student's Name _____ Date _____

Instructor's Name _____

SKILL   The dental assistant is responsible for preparation of equipment and supplies needed for appointments. Polycarboxylate cement, also known as zinc polycarboxylate, is used for permanent cementation and as an insulating base. There are several brands of polycarboxylate cement, and the cement comes in a powder/liquid form.

PERFORMANCE OBJECTIVE   The student will follow a routine procedure that meets the regulations and the protocol set forth by the dentist and regulatory agencies, keeping in mind that assistants' duties vary from state to state. The assistant may be evaluated by performance, statement, and/or combined responses and action. The dental assistant prepares and mixes the polycarboxylate materials to the desired consistency. The amount of materials dispensed depends on the size of restoration and the number of units involved.

	Self Evaluation	Student Evaluation	Possible Points	Instructor Evaluation	Comments
Equipment and Supplies					
1. Polycarboxylate powder and liquid and a dispenser for the powder			3		
2. Paper pad or glass slab			2		
3. Flexible stainless steel spatula			3		
4. 2 x 2 gauze sponge (moistened)			2		
5. Timer			2		
6. Plastic filling instrument			3		
Competency Steps					
1. Powder fluffed before dispensing with dispensing scoop.			3		
2. Powder measured and dispensed on one side of paper pad or glass slab.			3		
3. Uniform drops of liquid placed toward opposite side of powder (follow manufacturer's directions for appropriate powder/liquid ration).			3		
4. Incorporate three-fourths to all of powder into liquid			3		
A. Use folding motion while applying some pressure to wet all the powder			2		
B. Mix quickly until all powder is incorporated (liquid thick, harder to incorporate powder)			2		
5. Mix will be slightly more viscous than zinc phosphate cement and is glossy.			3		
6. Gather all cement up, wiping both sides of spatula.			2		
7. For luting consistency, mix will follow spatula up one inch.			3		

26-3 continued *(corresponds to textbook Procedure 26-4)*

	Self Evaluation	Student Evaluation	Possible Points	Instructor Evaluation	Comments
8. Base consistency, same amount of powder is used, but liquid ratio is decreased.			3		
A. Mix for base should be glossy			3		
B. Consistency is tacky and stiff			3		
9. Mix must be used immediately before it becomes dull and stringy.			3		
10. Cleanup done immediately			3		
A. Wipe spatula with wet 2 x 2 gauze			3		
B. Or soak spatula with dried cement in 10% sodium hydroxide solution			3		
C. Paper pad sheet removed, folded, and disposed			2		

TOTAL POINTS POSSIBLE   62

TOTAL POINTS POSSIBLE—2nd Attempt   60

TOTAL POINTS EARNED   _____

Points assigned reflect importance of step to meeting objective: Important = 1; Essential = 2; Critical = 3. Students will lose 2 points for repeated attempts. Failure results if any of the critical steps are omitted or performed incorrectly. If using a 100-point scale, determine score by dividing points earned by total points possible and multiplying the results by 100.

SCORE: _____

SKILL COMPETENCY ASSESSMENT

26-4 Mixing Glass Ionomer Cement *(corresponds to textbook Procedure 26-5)*

Student's Name _____ Date _____

Instructor's Name _____

SKILL The dental assistant is responsible for preparation of equipment and supplies needed for appointments. Glass ionomer cement is one of the newer cement systems. This cement is diverse in its applications, thus, there is more than one type of glass ionomer material. Glass ionomer cements come in numerous brands. It comes in powder/liquid, paste systems, syringes, and capsule forms. The glass ionomers come in both self-curing and light curing materials. The materials should be mixed quickly following manufacturer's directions because of the water content of the liquid. Water evaporation will affect the properties of the cement.

PERFORMANCE OBJECTIVE The student will follow a routine procedure that meets the regulations and the protocol set forth by the dentist and regulatory agencies, keeping in mind that assistants' duties vary from state to state. The assistant may be evaluated by performance, statement, and/or combined responses and action. This procedure is completed by the assistant for the dentist. The equipment and materials are prepared and mixed when the dentist indicates. The material must be used immediately when the mix is completed. This material requires the tooth to be clean of debris and dry, so the dental assistant should rinse and evacuate and then isolate the area before beginning to mix the cement.

	Self Evaluation	Student Evaluation	Possible Points	Instructor Evaluation	Comments
Equipment and Supplies					
1. Glass ionomer materials and appropriate dispensers			3		
2. Paper pad or cool glass slab			3		
3. Flexible stainless steel spatula			3		
4. 2 x 2 gauze sponge (moistened)			2		
5. Timer			2		
6. Plastic filling instrument			3		
Competency Steps					
1. Fluff powder before dispensing.			3		
2. Using recommended scoop, place appropriate number of scoops on paper pad or glass slab.			3		
3. Swirl liquid, then place specified amount of drops onto pad near powder (replace cap on liquid immediately to prevent evaporation).			3		
4. Divide powder into halves or thirds and then draw sections into liquid one at a time.			3		
5. Mix over small area until all powder is incorporated			3		
A. Luting consistency—creamy and glossy			3		
B. Base consistency—tacky and stiff			3		
6. Once cement has obtained final consistency:					
A. Wipe spatula off with 2 x 2 gauze			2		
B. Hold pad or glass slab under patient's chin			2		
C. Pass plastic filling instrument to dentist			3		

26-4 continued *(corresponds to textbook Procedure 26-5)*

	Self Evaluation	Student Evaluation	Possible Points	Instructor Evaluation	Comments
7. To clean up, remove top paper, fold, dispose of. Wipe instruments after use for easier cleanup.			3		
8. Glass ionomer capsules are activated by placement in "activator" or dispenser to break seal (allows powder and liquid to mix).			3		
9. Place capsules in amalgamator to mix (triturated) for specific amount of time (usually ten seconds—follow manufacturer's direction).			3		
10. Insert capsule in appropriate dispenser and pass to dentist for dispensing the material needed.			3		
11. To clean up, the capsule is discarded, and the activator and the dispenser are disinfected.			3		

TOTAL POINTS POSSIBLE   59

TOTAL POINTS POSSIBLE—2nd Attempt   57

TOTAL POINTS EARNED   _____

Points assigned reflect importance of step to meeting objective: Important = 1; Essential = 2; Critical = 3. Students will lose 2 points for repeated attempts. Failure results if any of the critical steps are omitted or performed incorrectly. If using a 100-point scale, determine score by dividing points earned by total points possible and multiplying the results by 100.

SCORE: _____

SKILL COMPETENCY ASSESSMENT

26-5 Mixing of Calcium Hydroxide Cement—Two-Paste System
(corresponds to textbook Procedure 26-6)

Student's Name _____ Date _____

Instructor's Name _____

SKILL The dental assistant is responsible for preparation of equipment and supplies needed for appointments. The two-paste system is mixed on a small paper pad with a metal spatula, an explorer, or a small ball-ended instrument. The base and the catalyst of the two-paste system come as a set and cannot be interchanged with other calcium hydroxide paste systems.

PERFORMANCE OBJECTIVE The student will follow a routine procedure that meets the regulations and the protocol set forth by the dentist and regulatory agencies, keeping in mind that assistants' duties vary from state to state. The assistant may be evaluated by performance, statement, and/or combined responses and action. This material is dispensed and mixed by the dental assistant. It is often the first step in restoring the cavity preparation.

	Self Evaluation	Student Evaluation	Possible Points	Instructor Evaluation	Comments
Equipment and Supplies					
1. Calcium hydrozide two-paste system			3		
2. Small paper pad			2		
3. Small ball-ended instrument or explorer			3		
4. 2 x 2 gauze sponge			2		
Competency Steps					
1. Dispense small, equal amounts of both catalyst and base onto paper pad.			3		
2. Wipe off ends of tubes, replace caps.			3		
3. Mix the two materials, using circular motion.			3		
4. Mix until materials are uniform color, within the ten to fifteen second mixing time.			3		
5. Use 2 x 2 gauze to remove excess material from mixing instrument.			3		
6. Pass instrument to dentist and hold paper pad close to patient's chin.			3		
7. Wipe instrument off with gauze for dentist between applications.			2		
8. Receive instrument, wipe it off, tear and fold the top page of paper pad, and dispose of it.			3		

TOTAL POINTS POSSIBLE	33	
TOTAL POINTS POSSIBLE—2nd Attempt	31	
TOTAL POINTS EARNED	_____	

Points assigned reflect importance of step to meeting objective: Important = 1; Essential = 2; Critical = 3. Students will lose 2 points for repeated attempts. Failure results if any of the critical steps are omitted or performed incorrectly. If using a 100-point scale, determine score by dividing points earned by total points possible and multiplying the results by 100.

SCORE: _____

SKILL COMPETENCY ASSESSMENT

26-6 Placing Resin Cement—Dual-Curing Technique
(corresponds to textbook Procedure 26-8)

Student's Name _____ Date _____

Instructor's Name _____

SKILL   The dental assistant is responsible for preparation of equipment and supplies needed for appointments. Resin cements may be supplied in a two-paste system, powder/liquid set, or syringe. The manufacturer may supply the acid-etch gel or liquid with the material. Some of these materials may be shaded to complement the translucency of the crown or inlay.

PERFORMANCE OBJECTIVE   The student will follow a routine procedure that meets the regulations and the protocol set forth by the dentist and regulatory agencies, keeping in mind that assistants' duties vary from state to state. The assistant may be evaluated by performance, statement, and/or combined responses and action. This procedure is prepared by the assistant for the dentist. The equipment and materials are prepared, and the material is mixed and passed to the dentist. Because this material is dual curing, a curing light and eye protection are needed.

	Self Evaluation	Student Evaluation	Possible Points	Instructor Evaluation	Comments
Equipment and Supplies					
1. Resin cement system			3		
2. Paper pad			2		
3. Stainless steel spatula			3		
4. Plastic filling instrument			3		
5. Curing light and protective shield or glasses			3		
6. 2 x 2 gauze sponges			2		
Competency Steps					
1. Clean and dry tooth and isolate area with cotton rolls.			3		
2. Pass etchant to dentist.			3		
3. Wait required time for etchant.			3		
4. Rinse thoroughly.			3		
5. Dry tooth.			3		
6. Dispense and mix the two components together to a homogeneous, creamy mixture.			3		
7. Hold pad close to patient and pass placement instrument (dentist places material on tooth and restoration).			3		
8. Hold 2 x 2 gauze to remove any excess materials.			2		
9. Receive placement instrument and prepare curing light.			3		
10. Use protective shield when curing light activated (either dentist or assistant holds light).			3		

26-6 continued *(corresponds to textbook Procedure 26-8)*

	Self Evaluation	Student Evaluation	Possible Points	Instructor Evaluation	Comments
11. Cleanup is done immediately (any excess cement is wiped off instruments and disposable items discarded).			3		

TOTAL POINTS POSSIBLE	48	
TOTAL POINTS POSSIBLE—2nd Attempt	46	
TOTAL POINTS EARNED	_____	

Points assigned reflect importance of step to meeting objective: Important = 1; Essential = 2; Critical = 3. Students will lose 2 points for repeated attempts. Failure results if any of the critical steps are omitted or performed incorrectly. If using a 100-point scale, determine score by dividing points earned by total points possible and multiplying the results by 100.

SCORE: _____

SKILL COMPETENCY ASSESSMENT

26-7 Placing Etchant *(corresponds to textbook Procedure 26-9)*

Student's Name _____ Date _____

Instructor's Name _____

SKILL   The dental assistant is responsible for preparation of equipment and supplies needed for appointments. Adhesion of dental materials to enamel is accomplished by acid etching with phosphoric acid. This solution alters the surface of the enamel and creates microscopic undercuts between the enamel rod. Unfilled resin bonding agents penetrate into these undercuts and mechanically lock into them. The restorative material then bonds to this layer and becomes a solid unit.

PERFORMANCE OBJECTIVE   The student will follow a routine procedure that meets the regulations and the protocol set forth by the dentist and regulatory agencies, keeping in mind that assistants' duties vary from state to state. The assistant may be evaluated by performance, statement and/or combined responses and action. The dental assistant prepares the materials and isolates the area. The dentist will place the etchant. When the allotted time has passed the assistant thoroughly rinses the tooth.

	Self Evaluation	Student Evaluation	Possible Points	Instructor Evaluation	Comments
Equipment and Supplies					
1. Acid etchant usually a 30 to 40% solution			3		
2. Isolation materials—rubber dam or cotton rolls			3		
3. Applicator—syringe, cotton pellets, small applicator tips			3		
4. Dappen dish			2		
5. Air-water syringe			2		
6. Timer			2		
Competency Steps					
1. Isolate the area.			3		
2. Clean surface thoroughly.			3		
3. Prepare etchant applicator or syringe.			3		
4. Place etchant on surface for fifteen to thirty seconds (follow manufacturer's direction).			3		
5. When time is up, rinse tooth for fifteen to twenty seconds with air-water syringe and evacuate thoroughly for ten to twenty seconds.			3		
6. Etched surface should have a frosty appearance.			3		
7. Until the bonding is completed, surface must be kept isolated and dry (if saliva or other fluids contact surface, etching process must be repeated).			3		

TOTAL POINTS POSSIBLE   36

TOTAL POINTS POSSIBLE—2nd Attempt   34

TOTAL POINTS EARNED   _____

Points assigned reflect importance of step to meeting objective: Important = 1; Essential = 2; Critical = 3. Students will lose 2 points for repeated attempts. Failure results if any of the critical steps are omitted or performed incorrectly. If using a 100-point scale, determine score by dividing points earned by total points possible and multiplying the results by 100.

SCORE: _____

SKILL COMPETENCY ASSESSMENT

26-8 Placing Bonding Agent *(corresponds to textbook Procedure 26-10)*

Student's Name _____ Date _____

Instructor's Name _____

SKILL   The dental assistant is responsible for preparation of equipment and supplies needed for appointments. The current dentin bonding materials use an etchant to remove the smear layer because the smear layer is not firmly attached and is unreliable. When the smear layer is removed, the adhesives can achieve a mechanical bond with the dentin. Many of the bonding agents are suitable for both enamel and dentin surfaces because of the application of the acid etchant.

PERFORMANCE OBJECTIVE   The student will follow a routine procedure that meets the regulations and the protocol set forth by the dentist and regulatory agencies, keeping in mind that assistants' duties vary from state to state. The assistant may be evaluated by performance, statement, and/or combined responses and action. Steps in the application of bonding agents vary with manufacturers, so follow the directions that come with the product. The dental assistant prepares the materials for each step and keeps the area dry and free of debris.

	Self Evaluation	Student Evaluation	Possible Points	Instructor Evaluation	Comments
Equipment and Supplies					
1. Bonding system that contains acid etchant, primer or conditioner, adhesive material			3		
2. Applicators (disposable tips or brushes)			3		
3. Dappen dish			2		
4. Isolation means			3		
5. Air-water syringe			2		
6. Curing light and shield			3		
7. Timer			2		
Competency Steps					
1. Cavity preparation must be clean (free of debris, sometimes cavity cleaners used).			3		
2. If cavity preparation is near pulp, place calcium hydroxide or glass ionomer lining cement over area.			3		
3. Etchant placed on surface (fifteen to twenty seconds) (first on enamel and then dentin).			3		
4. Rinse tooth as soon as time is up. Continue to rinse for five to ten seconds. Move quickly to prevent bacterial contamination of dentin.			3		
5. Primer or conditioner is placed with brush or applicator. If bonding involves both enamel and dentin, primer step included ("wets" dentin, penetrates into dentin tubules).			3		
6. Bonding resin applied.			3		
7. Curing light used to harden material.			3		

26-8 continued *(corresponds to textbook Procedure 26-10)*

	Self Evaluation	Student Evaluation	Possible Points	Instructor Evaluation	Comments
8. Clean up—dispose of applicator tips or brushes.			2		

TOTAL POINTS POSSIBLE   41

TOTAL POINTS POSSIBLE—2nd Attempt   39

TOTAL POINTS EARNED   _____

Points assigned reflect importance of step to meeting objective: Important = 1; Essential = 2; Critical = 3. Students will lose 2 points for repeated attempts. Failure results if any of the critical steps are omitted or performed incorrectly. If using a 100-point scale, determine score by dividing points earned by total points possible and multiplying the results by 100.

SCORE: _____

SKILL COMPETENCY ASSESSMENT

| 26-9 Amalgam Restoration—Class II (*corresponds to textbook Procedure 26-12*)

Student's Name _____ Date _____

Instructor's Name _____

SKILL The dental assistant is responsible for preparation of equipment and supplies needed for appointments. The sequence of procedure is for a complete amalgam restoration. The steps include administrating anesthetic, placing the rubber dam, placing liners and bases, assembling the matrix and wedge, mixing, placing, condensing, and finishing the amalgam restoration.

PERFORMANCE OBJECTIVE The student will follow a routine procedure that meets the regulations and the protocol set forth by the dentist and regulatory agencies, keeping in mind that assistants' duties vary from state to state. The assistant may be evaluated by performance, statement, and/or combined responses and action. The dental assistant assists the dentist throughout the procedure.

   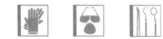

	Self Evaluation	Student Evaluation	Possible Points	Instructor Evaluation	Comments
Equipment and Supplies					
1. Basic setup: mouth mirror, explorer, cotton pliers			3		
2. Air-water syringe tip, HVE tip, and saliva ejector			3		
3. Cotton rolls, gauze sponges, pellets, cotton-tip applicators, and floss			3		
4. Topical and local anesthetic setup			3		
5. Rubber dam setup			3		
6. High- and low-speed handpieces			3		
7. Assortment of dental burs			3		
8. Spoon excavator			2		
9. Hand cutting instruments (hatches, chisels, hoes, gingival margin trimmers)			3		
10. Base, liner, varnish			3		
11. Paper pad, cement spatula, and placement instrument			3		
12. Matrix retainer, matrix bands, and wedges			3		
13. Locking pliers or hemostat			2		
14. Amalgam capsules			3		
15. Amalgam well			2		
16. Amalgam carrier and condensers			3		
17. Amalgamator			3		
18. Carving instruments			3		
19. Articulating paper and forceps			3		
Competency Steps					
1. Greet and prepare patient for procedure.			3		
2. Assistant reviews medical history.			3		

26-9 continued *(corresponds to textbook Procedure 26-12)*

	Self Evaluation	Student Evaluation	Possible Points	Instructor Evaluation	Comments
Anesthetic					
1. Prepare topical for local anesthetic.			2		
2. Assistant dries injection site and applies topical anesthetic (EF).			3		
3. Assistant prepares syringe and summons dentist.			2		
4. Assistant passes mirror, explorer to dentist (examine tooth before beginning procedure).			3		
5. When dentist is ready, assistant passes 2 x 2 gauze in one hand, syringe in other.			3		
6. Dentist replaces needle cap and places syringe on tray.			3		
7. Assistant rinses and evacuates patient's mouth (after injection).			3		
Dental Dam Placement					
8. Dental dam placement (EF)			3		
or					
9. Assistant prepares rubber dam materials and equipment, assists dentist in placement.			3		
Cavity Preparation					
1. Assistant passes mouth mirror and high-speed handpiece with a bur.			3		
2. Assistant positions HVE tip and maintains visibility throughout procedure.			3		
3. Assistant maintains cheek and tongue retraction.			3		
4. Assistant keeps mirror clear with air-water syringe while evacuating site.			3		
5. Assistant passes and receives instruments at dentist's signal (such as explorer, excavator, hatches, hoes, angle formers, gingival margin trimmers, and chisels).			3		
Cavity Liner and Cement Base Placement (EF)					
1. When preparation is finished, assistant passes a cotton pellet for cavity cleaning inside preparation.			3		
2. Area is rinsed and dried.			3		
3. At dentist direction, assistant mixes cavity liner.			3		
4. Prepares varnish.			2		
5. Prepares base.			3		
6. Passes them to dentist for placement.			3		
7. Light cured materials					
A. Assistant holds light tip near material			3		
B. Also holds protective shield			3		
C. Activates the light to cure material			3		

26-9 **continued** *(corresponds to textbook Procedure 26-12)*

	Self Evaluation	Student Evaluation	Possible Points	Instructor Evaluation	Comments
Placement of the Matrix and Wedge (EF)					
1. Assistant assembles matrix retainer and band (correct position for tooth being restored).			3		
2. Passes assembled matrix and band to dentist.			3		
3. After matrix placed, passes wedge in cotton pliers or hemostat.			3		
4. Dentist places wedge.			3		
Amalgam Placement					
1. Assistant prepares amalgam capsule when dentist ready (twist cap, squeeze capsule together, or place into activator, then place into amalgamator).			3		
2. Amalgamator set for specific type amalgam and size of mix.			3		
3. Amalgam material mixed.			3		
4. Assistant removes capsule from amalgamator and places amalgam into well or dappen dish.			3		
5. Amalgam loaded into carrier (double ended; load both ends).			3		
6. Loaded carrier passed to dentist.			3		
7. Alternately carrier and condenser exchanged (some offices, assistant loads carrier and places amalgam as dentist directs).			3		
8. After last exchange, assistant passes explorer (amalgam is loosened from matrix band).			3		
9. Assistant cleans up scrap amalgam from carrier and well and places them in sealed container.			3		
Remove the Matrix and Carve the Restoration					
1. Assistant receives explorer and passes carving and finishing instruments at dentist's signal. Assistant operates the HVE tip near site to evacuate any amalgam particles.			3 3		
2. After dentist completes preliminary carving, assistant passes cotton pliers to remove wedge.			3		
3. Assistant receives pliers and matrix retainer.			3		
4. Cotton pliers may be used again to remove band.			3		
5. Assistant receives cotton pliers and band and passes carver.			3		
Dental Dam Removal (EF) (rubber dam carefully removed at this time)					
1. Assistant passes clamp forceps.			3		
2. Assistant receives forceps with clamp.			3		
3. Passes scissors (cut interseptal dam).			3		

26-9 continued *(corresponds to textbook Procedure 26-12)*

	Self Evaluation	Student Evaluation	Possible Points	Instructor Evaluation	Comments
4. Assistant receives scissors, frame, napkin, and dam material.			3		
5. Assistant rinses and evacuates patient's mouth.			3		
Evaluation of Patient's Bite					
1. Assistant dries area and passes articulating paper (already assembled in forceps to pass to dentist).			3		
2. Dentist may instruct assistant to place paper over restoration.			2		
3. Patient will be instructed to gently tap teeth together.			2		
4. Additional carving may be continued until dentist is satisfied patient is comfortable.			2		
Dismiss the Patient					
1. Restoration is wiped off with wet cotton roll (to remove any blue marks left by articulating paper).			2		
2. Assistant rinses and evacuates the patient's mouth thoroughly.			3		
3. Cleans any debris from patient's face.			2		
4. Patient is cautioned not to chew on side of restoration for a few hours.			3		
5. Patient is dismissed.			2		

TOTAL POINTS POSSIBLE   219

TOTAL POINTS POSSIBLE—2nd Attempt   217

TOTAL POINTS EARNED   _____

Points assigned reflect importance of step to meeting objective: Important = 1; Essential = 2; Critical = 3. Students will lose 2 points for repeated attempts. Failure results if any of the critical steps are omitted or performed incorrectly. If using a 100-point scale, determine score by dividing points earned by total points possible and multiplying the results by 100.

SCORE: _____

SKILL COMPETENCY ASSESSMENT

26-10 Composite Restoration—Class III *(corresponds to textbook Procedure 26-13)*

Student's Name _____ Date _____

Instructor's Name _____

SKILL   The dental assistant is responsible for preparation of equipment and supplies needed for appointments. These direct restorative materials are inserted into the cavity preparation and then self-cured, light cured, or dual cured. They come in syringes or single application cartridges (compules) and have a variety of shades or shade modifiers. The location and the size of the cavity will determine which material the dentist chooses.

PERFORMANCE OBJECTIVE   The student will follow a routine procedure that meets the regulations and the protocol set forth by the dentist and regulatory agencies, keeping in mind that assistants' duties vary from state to state. The assistant may be evaluated by performance, statement, and/or combined responses and action. The dental assistant assists the dentist throughout the procedure.

	Self Evaluation	Student Evaluation	Possible Points	Instructor Evaluation	Comments
Equipment and Supplies					
1. Basic setup: mouth mirror, explorer, cotton pliers			3		
2. Air-water syringe tip, HVE tip, and saliva ejector			3		
3. Cotton rolls, gauze sponges, cotton pellets, cotton-tip applicators, and floss			3		
4. Topical and local anesthetic setup			3		
5. Rubber dam setup			3		
6. High- and low-speed handpieces			3		
7. Assortment of dental burs (including diamond and cutting burs)			3		
8. Spoon excavator			2		
9. Hand cutting instruments (dentist's choice may include binangle chisel and Wedelstaedt chisel)			3		
10. Base and liner with mixing materials and placement instruments			3		
11. Etchant and applicator, if necessary (usually comes with composite system)			3		
12. Primer (usually comes with composite system)			3		
13. Composite materials, including shade guide			3		
14. Composite placement instrument (plastic filling instrument)			3		
15. Curing light with protective shield			3		
16. Celluloid matrix strip and wedges			3		
17. Locking pliers or hemostat			3		
18. Finishing burs or diamonds			3		
19. #12 scalpel			3		
20. Abrasive strips			3		
21. Polishing discs			3		

26-10 continued *(corresponds to textbook Procedure 26-13)*

	Self Evaluation	Student Evaluation	Possible Points	Instructor Evaluation	Comments
22. Lubricant			2		
23. Articulating paper and forceps			3		
Competency Steps					
1. Greet and prepare patient for procedure (patient is seated).			3		
2. Assistant reviews medical history.			3		
Anesthetic					
1. Prepare topical for local anesthetic (have patient rinse mouth).			3		
2. Assistant dries injection site and applies topical anesthetic (EF).			3		
3. Assistant prepares syringe and summons dentist.			2		
4. Assistant removes topical anesthetic applicator, and transfers mirror and explorer to dentist.			3		
5. When dentist ready, assistant passes 2 x 2 gauze in one hand, syringe in other.			3		
6. Dentist replaces needle cap and places syringe on tray.			3		
7. After injection, assistant rinses and evacuates patient's mouth.			3		
Determine shade					
1. Select shade under natural light.			3		
2. Combination of shades may be selected.			3		
3. Shade selection recorded on patient's chart.			3		
Dental Dam Placement					
1. Assistant places dental dam or prepares rubber dam materials and equipment for dentist.			3		
Cavity Preparation					
1. Assistant passes mouth mirror and high-speed handpiece with a bur.			3		
2. Assistant positions HVE tip and maintains visibility throughout procedure.			3		
3. Assistant maintains check and tongue retraction.			3		
4. Assistant keeps mirror clear with air-water syringe while evacuating site.			3		
5. At dentist's signal, assistant passes and receives instruments, such as: explorer, excavator, binangle chisel, wedelstaedt chisel, etc.			3		

26-10 continued *(corresponds to textbook Procedure 26-13)*

	Self Evaluation	Student Evaluation	Possible Points	Instructor Evaluation	Comments
6. May be directed to change the dentist's bur.			3		
Cavity protection: Cavity liner and cement base placement (EF)					
1. When preparation is finished, assistant passes a cotton pellet for cavity cleaning inside preparation			3		
2. Area is rinsed and dried.			3		
3. At dentist direction, assistant mixes cavity liner (determined by dentist base, liner).			3		
4. Assistant holds mixing pad, applicator, 2 x 2 gauze near patient's chin (after each application, wipes instrument).			3		
5. Passes them to dentist for placement.			3		
6. Light cured materials					
A. Assistant holds light tip near material			3		
B. Also holds protective shield			3		
C. Activates the light to cure material			3		
Application of the Etchant					
1. Assistant passes brush or applicator tip containing acid etchant material to dentist.			3		
2. Etchant is rinsed thoroughly after recommended time.			3		
Matrix and Wedge					
1. Celluloid matrix strip placed by dentist.			2		
2. Passes matrix to dentist.			2		
3. After matrix placed, passes wedge in cotton pliers or hemostat (plastic wedge if needed).			3		
4. Dentist places wedge.			3		
Placing the Bonding Material					
1. Bonding material placed according to manufacturer's directions.			3		
2. Bonding resins: primer or conditioner (placed before bonding material).			3		
Placement of the Composite					
1. Assistant prepares composite of choice.			3		
2. Syringe loaded with color-selected material.			3		
3. Syringe passed to dentist.			3		
4. Assistant passes filling instrument.			3		
5. Light cured material is placed in incremental layers.			3		

26-10 continued *(corresponds to textbook Procedure 26-13)*

	Self Evaluation	Student Evaluation	Possible Points	Instructor Evaluation	Comments
6. Within a few minutes, material begins to chemically set.			3		
Remove the Matrix and Carve the Restoration					
1. Assistant passes dentist cotton pliers to remove wedge and matrix strip.			3		
2. After receiving wedge and matrix strip, pass explorer.			3		
Finishing and Polishing					
1. Assistant passes the low-speed handpiece with finishing bur to dentist.			3		
2. Assistant uses air syringe while dentist uses handpiece.			3		
3. Assistant may need to change burs, finishing burs, diamonds, and abrasive disks.			3		
4. Abrasive strips may be needed to smooth interproximal areas.			3		
5. To smooth, polish points, disks, and cups.			3		
Dental Dam Removal (EF)					
1. Assistant passes clamp forceps.			3		
2. Assistant receives forceps with clamp.			3		
3. Passes scissors for cutting interseptal dam.			3		
4. Assistant receives scissors, frame, napkin, and dam material.			3		
5. Assistant rinses and evacuates patient's mouth.			3		
Evaluation of Patient's Bite					
1. Assistant dries area and passes articulating paper already assembled in forceps.			3		
2. Dentist may instruct assistant to place over restoration.			2		
3. Patient will be instructed to tap teeth together.			2		
4. Additional carving may be continued until dentist is satisfied patient is comfortable.			2		
Dismiss the Patient					
1. Restoration is wiped off with wet cotton roll (to remove any blue marks left by articulating paper).			2		
2. Assistant rinses and evacuates the patient's mouth thoroughly.			3		
3. Cleans any debris from patient's face.			2		

26-10 continued *(corresponds to textbook Procedure 26-13)*

	Self Evaluation	Student Evaluation	Possible Points	Instructor Evaluation	Comments
4. Patient is given postoperative instructions.			3		
5. Patient is dismissed.			2		

TOTAL POINTS POSSIBLE   244

TOTAL POINTS POSSIBLE—2nd Attempt   242

TOTAL POINTS EARNED   _____

Points assigned reflect importance of step to meeting objective: Important = 1; Essential = 2; Critical = 3. Students will lose 2 points for repeated attempts. Failure results if any of the critical steps are omitted or performed incorrectly. If using a 100-point scale, determine score by dividing points earned by total points possible and multiplying the results by 100.

SCORE: _____

Laboratory Materials and Techniques

OBJECTIVES

The student should strive to meet the following objectives and demonstrate an understanding of the facts and principles presented in this chapter:

1. Identify the materials used in the dental laboratory and perform the associated procedures.
2. Demonstrate the knowledge and skills needed to prepare, take, and remove alginate impressions and wax bites.
3. Demonstrate the knowledge and skills necessary to prepare reversible hydrocolloid impression material for the dentist.
4. Demonstrate the knowledge and skills necessary to prepare elastomeric impression materials such as polysulfide, silicone (polysiloxane and polyvinyl siloxanes), and polyether for the dentist.
5. Demonstrate the knowledge and skills necessary to use gypsum products such as Type I: Impression plaster, Type II: Laboratory or model plaster, Type III: Laboratory stone, Type IV: Die stone, and Type V: High-strength die stone.
6. Demonstrate the knowledge and skills necessary to pour and trim a patient's alginate impression (diagnostic cast).
7. Identify the use of a dental articulator for dental casts or study models.
8. Identify the different classifications and uses of waxes used in dentistry.
9. Demonstrate the knowledge and skills necessary to fabricate acrylic tray resin self-curing and light-curing custom trays, vacuum-formed, and thermoplastic custom trays.
10. Demonstrate the knowledge and skills necessary to contour prefabricated temporary crowns and to fabricate and fit custom temporary restorations.

SUMMARY

A number of basic functions in the dental laboratory are routinely performed by the dental assistant, such as pouring and trimming study models, fabricating custom trays, and fabricating provisional temporaries. To accomplish these procedures, the dental assistant must understand the materials that are used, the properties of each material, and the steps in each procedure. Any dental assistant who has skills in performing laboratory duties will be an asset to his or her employer. The better crossed-trained the dental team members are, the better the dental office functions.

KEY TERMS

accelerates	gel	polymer	sol
articulator	gypsum	polymerization	study models
calcination	homogenous	polysulfide	syneresis
catalyst	imbibition	reversible hydrocolloid	thermoplastic
distortion	irreversible hydrocolloid	silicones	undercuts
exothermic reaction	monomer		

EXERCISES AND ACTIVITIES

1. Alginate impressions make a _____ mold.
   A. negative   C. sol
   B. positive   D. agar-agar

2. Alginate is a generic name used for a group of _____ impression materials.
   A. reversible hydrocolloid
   B. irreversible hydrocolloid
   C. polysulfide
   D. gypsum

3. The disadvantages of alginates primarily come from the loss of accuracy due to atmospheric conditions. If an impression loses water content due to heat, dryness, or exposure to air, it causes shrinkage, a condition known as _____
   A. imbibition.
   B. an exothermic reaction.
   C. polymerization.
   D. syneresis.

4. If an impression takes on additional water and causing swelling, the impression will have a dimensional enlargement, known as _____
   A. calcination.
   B. syneresis.
   C. imbibition.
   D. an exothermic reaction.

5. All the elastomeric impression materials have a catalyst and base that are mixed together to start the chemical self-curing process. The process by which the catalyst and accelerator begin to cure is called _____
   A. an exothermic reaction.
   B. polymerization.
   C. distortion.
   D. calcination.

6. The elastomeric impression materials have a rubber-like quality and are used for areas that require precise duplication. _____ is a dimensional change in shape.
   A. Imbibition   C. Calcination
   B. Distortion   D. Syneresis

7. To start the chemical self-curing process, a _____ and base are mixed together.
   A. gel   C. resin
   B. sol   D. catalyst

8. Which of the following is not an elastomeric impression material? _____
   A. Silicone   C. Polyether
   B. Agar-agar   D. Polysulfide

9. Of the primary types of gypsum used in dentistry, which type is for model or laboratory plaster? _____
   A. Type I   C. Type III
   B. Type II   D. Type IV

10. _____ is an elastomeric impression material that is available in putty form for making a custom tray.
    A. Silicone   C. Polysulfide
    B. Polyether   D. Methacrylate

11. The strengths of gypsum products are determined by the _____ process and the water/powder ratio needed to incorporate the mixture.
    A. thermoplastic   C. polymerization
    B. exothermic   D. calcination

12. A(n) _____ holds models of the patient's teeth to maintain the patient's occlusion and represent his or her jaws.
    A. articulator   C. conditioner
    B. vacuum former   D. extruder

13. Utility wax is used to bead around trays to extend them. Which group of waxes would utility wax be classified with? _____
    A. Impression   C. Pattern
    B. Processing   D. Other

14. The most common material used to make custom trays is the self-curing acrylic tray resin. The catalyst liquid that mixes with the powder is called _____
    A. polymer.   C. monomer.
    B. base.   D. sol.

15. The self-curing acrylic material goes through several stages of curing. During one of the stages the material goes through a(n) _____ reaction, giving off a great deal of heat while setting.
    A. initial set   C. kneaded
    B. exothermic   D. thermoplastic

16. _____ are recessed areas in a model that make it impossible to seat or remove a custom tray properly.
    A. Spacers   C. Matrices
    B. Undercuts   D. Stops

17. What term means that a material becomes soft and pliable when exposed to heat? _____
    A. Exothermic   C. Imbibition
    B. Thermoplastic   D. Syneresis

18. A material that is uniformly mixed is called _____
    A. homogenous.   C. irreversible.
    B. exothermic.   D. thermoplastic.

19. Which of the following are advantages of reversible hydrocolloid? _____
    1. More accurate than alginate
    2. Comparatively economical after initial equipment purchase
    3. Can be used for impressions for crown and bridge construction
    4. Less equipment needed
    5. Less setting time required
    6. Not affected by atmospheric conditions

    A. 1, 4, 5
    B. 1, 2, 6
    C. 1, 2, 3
    D. 2, 3, 4

20. Which of the following equipment and supplies would indicate the taking of a polysulfide impression? _____
    1. Custom tray painted with adhesive
    2. Water measure
    3. Glass slab
    4. Two pastes, base and catalyst
    5. Rubber bowl
    6. Rigid laboratory spatulas

    A. 2, 3, 5
    B. 2, 3, 6
    C. 1, 4, 6
    D. 1, 2, 3

SKILL COMPETENCY ASSESSMENT

27-1 Preparing for an Alginate Impression

Student's Name _____ Date _____

Instructor's Name _____

SKILL   The dental assistant is responsible for preparation of equipment and supplies needed for appointments. Alginate is a generic name used for a group of irreversible hydrocolloid impression materials. One of the most common areas where alginate is used is in making diagnostic casts or study models. In some states, dental assistants are allowed to take the alginate impressions; in other states, the assistant can select the tray, mix the material, load the material into the tray, and pass the tray for the dentist to place in the patient's mouth.

PERFORMANCE OBJECTIVE   The student will follow a routine procedure that meets the regulations and the protocol set forth by the dentist and regulatory agencies, keeping in mind that assistants' duties vary from state to state. The assistant may be evaluated by performance, statement, and/or combined responses and action. This procedure is performed by the dental assistant in the states where it is allowed. The materials are prepared and the alginate impression is taken on the maxillary and mandibular arches.

	Self Evaluation	Student Evaluation	Possible Points	Instructor Evaluation	Comments
Equipment and Supplies					
1. Flexible spatula/broad blade or disposable spatula			3		
2. Flexible rubber bowl(s) or disposable bowl			3		
3. Alginate material with water and powder measuring devices			3		
4. Water			3		
5. Impression tray(s)			3		
Competency Steps					
Patient Preparation					
1. Health history reviewed.			3		
2. Patient seated in upright position with protective napkin in place.			3		
3. Mouth rinsed with water or mouth rinse (remove food debris and aid with thick saliva).			3		
4. Explain procedure to patient.			3		
5. Impressions trays are tried into the oral cavity to determine correct size.			3		
Material Preparation					
1. Wax placed around borders of impression trays if necessary (extend borders of tray for patient comfort).			3		
2. Impression water measured for mandibular model (water, room temperature, two calibrations).			3		
3. Water placed first into flexible mixing bowl.			3		
4. Fluff powder prior to opening canister (follow manufacturer's directions as indicated).			3		

27-1 continued

	Self Evaluation	Student Evaluation	Possible Points	Instructor Evaluation	Comments
5. Fill measure of powder by overfilling and then level off with spatula (accurate measure).			3		
6. Dispense two corresponding scoops into a second flexible rubber bowl.			3		
7. When ready, place the powder into water.			3		
8. Mix water and powder first with a stirring motion.			3		
9. Then mix by holding bowl in one hand, rotating bowl occasionally, using flat side of spatula to incorporate material through pressure against side of bowl: mixing Type I, fast set thirty to forty-five seconds, Type II, regular set, one minute.			3		
10. Upon completion, mixture should be homogenous and creamy.			3		
11. Once material is mixed correctly, load the tray _____ (mandibular, load both lingual sides, use flat side of blade to condense material firmly into tray—if necessary to smooth surface, with gloved hand moisten and smooth top).			3		

TOTAL POINTS POSSIBLE   63

TOTAL POINTS POSSIBLE—2nd Attempt   61

TOTAL POINTS EARNED   _____

Points assigned reflect importance of step to meeting objective: Important = 1; Essential = 2; Critical = 3. Students will lose 2 points for repeated attempts. Failure results if any of the critical steps are omitted or performed incorrectly. If using a 100-point scale, determine score by dividing points earned by total points possible and multiplying the results by 100.

SCORE: _____

SKILL COMPETENCY ASSESSMENT

27-2 Taking an Alginate Impression

Student's Name _____ Date _____

Instructor's Name _____

SKILL   The dental assistant is responsible for preparation of equipment and supplies needed for appointments. Alginate is a generic name used for a group of irreversible hydrocolloid impression materials. One of the most common areas where algi-nate is used is making diagnostic casts or study models. In some states, dental assistants are allowed to take the alginate impres-sions; in other states, the assistant can select the tray, mix the material, load the material into the tray, and pass the tray for the dentist to place in the patient's mouth.

PERFORMANCE OBJECTIVE   The student will follow a routine procedure that meets the regulations and the protocol set forth by the dentist and regulatory agencies, keeping in mind that assistants' duties vary from state to state. The assistant may be evaluated by performance, statement, and/or combined responses and action. This procedure is performed by the dental assistant in the states where it is allowed. The materials are prepared and the alginate impression is taken on the maxillary and mandibular arches.

	Self Evaluation	Student Evaluation	Possible Points	Instructor Evaluation	Comments
Equipment and Supplies					
1. Flexible spatula/broad blade or dis-posable spatula			3		
2. Flexible rubber bowl(s) or disposable bowl			3		
3. Alginate material with water and powder measuring devices			3		
4. Water			3		
5. Impression tray(s)			3		
Competency Steps					
1. Facing patient, retract the right cheek of patient slightly.			3		
2. Use excess alginate material to rub onto occlusal surfaces of teeth to obtain more accurate anatomy.			3		
3. Invert impression tray so material is toward teeth.			3		
4. Turn tray so it passes through lip opening, with one side of tray entering first. Using other hand, retract opposite corner of mouth.			3		
5. When tray is completely in patient's mouth, center it above teeth.			3		
6. Lower tray onto teeth, placing posterior area down first, leaving impression tray slightly anterior.			3		
7. Have patient raise the tongue and move it side to side to ensure that lingual aspect of alveolar process will be defined in impression.			3		
8. Pull out lip from center with other hand.			3		

27-2 continued

	Self Evaluation	Student Evaluation	Possible Points	Instructor Evaluation	Comments
9. Finish placing impression tray down and, as it is done, push slightly toward the posterior area with tray (pushing impression material needed in anterior vestibule area—observe lip is out of the way).			3		
10. Allow lip to cover tray (lip positioned close to handle portion of tray).			3		
11. Hold tray in patient's mouth with two fingers on back of tray, one on right side, one on left side until set—material should feel firm and not change shape when touched (check excess material to determine set, sides of bowl, edges of impression tray).			3		
12. The maxillary alginate impression is loaded from posterior (allows to fill tray without voids).			3		
13. Take small amount of alginate from palate area (prevents impression material from going down patient's throat after insertion).			3		
14. Place maxillary tray into patient's mouth (turning tray so it passes through lip opening with one side of tray entering first, using other hand to retract opposite corner of mouth).			3		
15. Raise tray to maxillary arch and hold out lip prior to seating tray in place.			3		
16. Hold tray in position as in mandibular until the material is set in the bowl.			3		

TOTAL POINTS POSSIBLE   63

TOTAL POINTS POSSIBLE—2nd Attempt   61

TOTAL POINTS EARNED   _____

Points assigned reflect importance of step to meeting objective: Important = 1; Essential = 2; Critical = 3. Students will lose 2 points for repeated attempts. Failure results if any of the critical steps are omitted or performed incorrectly. If using a 100-point scale, determine score by dividing points earned by total points possible and multiplying the results by 100.

SCORE: _____

SKILL COMPETENCY ASSESSMENT

27-3 Removing the Alginate Impression

Student's Name _____ Date _____

Instructor's Name _____

SKILL   The dental assistant is responsible for preparation of equipment and supplies needed for appointments. Alginate is a generic name used for a group of irreversible hydrocolloid impression materials. One of the most common areas where alginate is used is in making diagnostic casts or study models. In some states, dental assistants are allowed to take the alginate impressions; in other states, the assistant can select the tray, mix the material, load the material into the tray, and pass the tray for the dentist to place in the patient's mouth.

PERFORMANCE OBJECTIVE   The student will follow a routine procedure that meets the regulations and the protocol set forth by the dentist and regulatory agencies, keeping in mind that assistants' duties vary from state to state. The assistant may be evaluated by performance, statement, and/or combined responses and action. This procedure is performed by the dental assistant in the states where it is allowed. The materials are prepared and the alginate impression is taken on the maxillary and mandibular arches.

	Self Evaluation	Student Evaluation	Possible Points	Instructor Evaluation	Comments
Equipment and Supplies					
1. Flexible spatula/broad blade or disposable spatula			3		
2. Flexible rubber bowl(s) or disposable bowl			3		
3. Alginate material with water and powder measuring devices			3		
4. Water			3		
5. Impression tray(s)			3		
Competency Steps					
1. When material is completely set, remove it from mouth (first loosening tissue of lips and cheek, around periphery, with fingers break suction-like seal).			3		
2. Place fingers of opposing hand on opposite arch to protect adjacent arch as tray is now removed.			3		
3. Remove tray in an upward or downward motion (depending on arch) with a quick snap.			3		
4. Turn tray to side to allow it to be removed from oral cavity.			3		
5. Remove any excess alginate material from patient's mouth.			2		
6. Rinse, evacuate, and have patient rinse out.			3		
7. Check patient's face for any excess alginate material. If present, give patient a tissue and mirror to remove material.			2		
8. Check impression for accuracy.			3		

27-3 continued

	Self Evaluation	Student Evaluation	Possible Points	Instructor Evaluation	Comments
9. Rinse impression gently with water to remove saliva or blood.			3		
10. Spray with approved surface disinfectant. If time lapse (maximum of twenty minutes) prior to pouring, wrap alginate in air-tight container and label with patient's name.			3		

TOTAL POINTS POSSIBLE   43

TOTAL POINTS POSSIBLE—2nd Attempt   41

TOTAL POINTS EARNED   _____

Points assigned reflect importance of step to meeting objective: Important = 1; Essential = 2; Critical = 3. Students will lose 2 points for repeated attempts. Failure results if any of the critical steps are omitted or performed incorrectly. If using a 100-point scale, determine score by dividing points earned by total points possible and multiplying the results by 100.

SCORE: _____

SKILL COMPETENCY ASSESSMENT

27-4 Disinfecting Alginate Impressions

Student's Name _____ Date _____

Instructor's Name _____

SKILL   The dental assistant is responsible for preparation of equipment and supplies needed for appointments. Alginate is a generic name used for a group of irreversible hydrocolloid impression materials. One of the most common areas where alginate is used is in making diagnostic casts or study models. In some states, dental assistants are allowed to take the alginate impressions; in other states, the assistant can select the tray, mix the material, load the material into the tray, and pass the tray for the dentist to place in the patient's mouth.

PERFORMANCE OBJECTIVE   The student will follow a routine procedure that meets the regulations and the protocol set forth by the dentist and regulatory agencies, keeping in mind that assistants' duties vary from state to state. The assistant may be evaluated by performance, statement, and/or combined responses and action. This procedure is performed by the dental assistant immediately after removing the alginate impressions from the patient's mouth and caring for the patient.

	Self Evaluation	Student Evaluation	Possible Points	Instructor Evaluation	Comments
Equipment and Supplies					
1. Approved disinfectant			3		
2. Covered container			3		
Competency Steps					
1. Impressions are rinsed gently under tap water to remove any debris, blood, or saliva.			3		
2. Impressions are sprayed with an approved disinfectant.			3		
3. Place impressions in covered container if not pouring immediately.			3		
4. Label container with patient's name.			3		
TOTAL POINTS POSSIBLE			27		
TOTAL POINTS POSSIBLE—2nd Attempt			25		
TOTAL POINTS EARNED			_____		

Points assigned reflect importance of step to meeting objective: Important = 1; Essential = 2; Critical = 3. Students will lose 2 points for repeated attempts. Failure results if any of the critical steps are omitted or performed incorrectly. If using a 100-point scale, determine score by dividing points earned by total points possible and multiplying the results by 100.

SCORE: _____

SKILL COMPETENCY ASSESSMENT

27-5 Taking a Bite Registration

Student's Name _____ Date _____

Instructor's Name _____

SKILL   The dental assistant is responsible for preparation of equipment and supplies needed for appointments. A wax bite registration is taken to establish the relationship between the maxillary and the mandibular teeth. Normally wax that is formed in a horseshoe shape is used, but the flat sheet of utility wax can be used as well. It is softened using warm water and then placed on the mandibular arch of the patient.

PERFORMANCE OBJECTIVE   The student will follow a routine procedure that meets the regulations and the protocol set forth by the dentist and regulatory agencies, keeping in mind that assistants' duties vary from state to state. The assistant may be evaluated by performance, statement, and/or combined responses and action. This procedure is performed by the dental assistant under the direction of the dentist or by the dentist with the dental assistant assisting.

	Self Evaluation	Student Evaluation	Possible Points	Instructor Evaluation	Comments
Equipment and Supplies					
1. Bite registration wax or wax horseshoe or polysiloxane and extruder gun and disposable tips			3		
2. Laboratory knife			3		
3. Warm water or torch			3		
Competency Steps					
1. Patient remains in upright position after impressions are taken (patient napkin in place).			3		
2. Procedure is explained to patient.			3		
3. Bite registration wax is tried in to determine correct length. Adjust and trim as needed with laboratory knife.			3		
4. Patient is instructed to practice biting to establish occlusion.			3		
5. Bite registration wax is heated (warm water or torch to soften).			3		
6. Wax is placed on mandibular occlusal surface of patient.			3		
7. Patient is instructed to gently bite together in the correct occlusion.			3		
8. Wax will cool (one to two minutes) while patient keeps teeth together in occlusion.			3		
9. Wax is then gently removed without distortion.			3		

27-5 continued

	Self Evaluation	Student Evaluation	Possible Points	Instructor Evaluation	Comments
10. Wax or polysiloxane bite registration is labeled and stored for use during trimming of diagnostic casts (study models).			3		

TOTAL POINTS POSSIBLE   39

TOTAL POINTS POSSIBLE—2nd Attempt   37

TOTAL POINTS EARNED   _____

Points assigned reflect importance of step to meeting objective: Important = 1; Essential = 2; Critical = 3. Students will lose 2 points for repeated attempts. Failure results if any of the critical steps are omitted or performed incorrectly. If using a 100-point scale, determine score by dividing points earned by total points possible and multiplying the results by 100.

SCORE: _____

SKILL COMPETENCY ASSESSMENT

27-6 Taking a Polysulfide Impression

Student's Name _____ Date _____

Instructor's Name _____

SKILL   The dental assistant is responsible for preparation of equipment and supplies needed for appointments. Polysulfide impression materials are supplied in two pastes, a base and a catalyst. These pastes can be purchased as light (syringe material), regular, heavy, and extra heavy (tray material). Ten minutes is required from the start of the mix to the setting of the material prior to removal from the patient's mouth. Knowledge of materials and factors that can slightly accelerate or shorten are critical to use.

PERFORMANCE OBJECTIVE   The student will follow a routine procedure that meets the regulations and the protocol set forth by the dentist and regulatory agencies, keeping in mind that assistants' duties vary from state to state. The assistant may be evaluated by performance, statement, and/or combined responses and action. This procedure is performed by the dentist with the dental assistant assisting. Polysulfide is a material used in taking final impressions where extreme accuracy is required.

STANDARD PRECAUTIONS   This can be a four- or six-handed procedure. All auxiliaries involved should wear some protection over clothing.

	Self Evaluation	Student Evaluation	Possible Points	Instructor Evaluation	Comments
Equipment and Supplies					
1. Two rigid, tapered, laboratory spatulas			3		
2. Paper pad, provided by the manufacturer			3		
3. Two pastes each from same manufacturer			3		
A. Two syringes, two trays—base and accelerator of syringe			3		
B. Base and accelerator of tray material			3		
4. Impression syringe with tip in place and plunger out of cylinder			3		
5. Custom tray that has been painted with corresponding adhesive and permitted to dry			3		
Competency Steps					
1. Health history reviewed.			3		
2. Patient seated in upright position with patient napkin in place and large throw over clothes.			3		
3. Mouth rinsed with water or mouth rinse (remove any food debris, aid removing thick saliva).			3		
4. Procedure explained to patient.			3		
5. Material mixed concurrently by two individuals (syringe material mixed slightly ahead of tray material; determine who will mix which parts).			3		
6. Dispense accelerator onto pad in long, even line about four inches (more material, more lines, wipe end of tube before placing lid back on).			3		
7. Dispense base onto pad in long, even line same length as accelerator (additional lines can be added, not to touch accelerator until operator wants mix process to begin—polymerization).			3		

27-6 continued

	Self Evaluation	Student Evaluation	Possible Points	Instructor Evaluation	Comments
8. Mixing materials:					
A. First, syringe material, mixes accelerator into base material, spatulate the pastes together with broad sweeps			3		
B. After a minute has lapsed, the individual mixing the tray material begins—same process			3		
9. When mix is homogenous, it is completely mixed (without brown or white streaks—takes forty-five seconds to a minute).			3		
10. Impression syringe:					
A. Load syringe material into impression syringe (fill back portion of barrel, pushing syringe over material repeatedly to force material into chamber)			3		
B. Place plunger into syringe (wipe edges quickly)			3		
C. Extrude material slightly to ensure it works			3		
D. Pass to dentist			3		
11. Tray material:					
A. Mixed same consistency, same time frame			3		
B. Material picked up by spatula and loaded into impression tray and spread evenly			3		
C. Tray passed to dentist after syringe used			3		
D. Mix and loading must be completed within four minutes			3		
12. Impression must remain in patient's mouth six minutes to achieve final set (held by operator or dental assistant).			3		
13. Cleanup accomplished after material has reached rubber stage—peels off spatula (remove top sheet of paper pad, throw away paper and disposable syringe, sterilize spatula).			3		
14. Removal of tray done in much same manner as alginate. Quick snap, releasing seal and taking care to protect opposing teeth.			3		

TOTAL POINTS POSSIBLE   81

TOTAL POINTS POSSIBLE—2nd Attempt   79

TOTAL POINTS EARNED   _____

Points assigned reflect importance of step to meeting objective: Important = 1; Essential = 2; Critical = 3. Students will lose 2 points for repeated attempts. Failure results if any of the critical steps are omitted or performed incorrectly. If using a 100-point scale, determine score by dividing points earned by total points possible and multiplying the results by 100.

SCORE: _____

SKILL COMPETENCY ASSESSMENT

27-7 Pouring an Alginate Impression for a Study Model
(corresponds to textbook Procedure 27-9)

Student's Name _____ Date _____

Instructor's Name _____

SKILL The dental assistant is responsible for preparation of equipment and supplies needed for appointments. Several different gypsum materials are used when pouring up an impression to make a model. It is important to identify the application for the material prior to determining the type of gypsum product to use. Plaster is a white stone (plaster of paris).

PERFORMANCE OBJECTIVE The student will follow a routine procedure that meets the regulations and the protocol set forth by the dentist and regulatory agencies, keeping in mind that assistants' duties vary from state to state. The assistant may be evaluated by performance, statement, and/or combined responses and action. This procedure is performed by the dental assistant in the dental laboratory immediately after mixing the plaster.

	Self Evaluation	Student Evaluation	Possible Points	Instructor Evaluation	Comments
Equipment and Supplies					
1. Metal spatula (stiff blade with rounded end) or disposable spatula			3		
2. Mixed plaster from Procedure 27-8			3		
3. Vibrator with paper towel or plastic cover on platform			3		
Competency Steps					
1. Use vibrator at low or medium (impression ready to pour, excess moisture removed, laboratory knife used to eliminate excess impression material—not to hamper pouring).			3		
2. Hold impression by handle, tray portion on platform of vibrator, allow small amount of plaster touch most distal surface of one side of arch in impression.			3		
3. Continue to add small increments of plaster in same area (plaster flows around toward anterior teeth and to other side of arch).			3		
4. Continue adding plaster until it flows out the other side of impression and fills the anatomic portion of model (rotate impression around platform of vibrator to allow material to travel around arch).			3		
5. After anatomy portion is filled with plaster, larger increments can be used to fill entire impression, off the vibrator.			3		
6. When filled, place lightly on vibrator to coalesce.			3		

27-7 continued *(corresponds to textbook Procedure 27-9)*

	Self Evaluation	Student Evaluation	Possible Points	Instructor Evaluation	Comments
7. If a two-pour method is used, small blobs should be left on top of plaster.			3		

TOTAL POINTS POSSIBLE   30

TOTAL POINTS POSSIBLE—2nd Attempt 28

TOTAL POINTS EARNED   _____

Points assigned reflect importance of step to meeting objective: Important = 1; Essential = 2; Critical = 3. Students will lose 2 points for repeated attempts. Failure results if any of the critical steps are omitted or performed incorrectly. If using a 100-point scale, determine score by dividing points earned by total points possible and multiplying the results by 100.

SCORE: _____

SKILL COMPETENCY ASSESSMENT

27-8 Trimming Diagnostic Casts/Study Models *(corresponds to textbook Procedure 27-12)*

Student's Name _____ Date _____

Instructor's Name _____

SKILL   The dental assistant is responsible for preparation of equipment and supplies needed for appointments. The diagnostic casts (study models) are used to present the case to the patient. It is important that these have an attractive appearance.

PERFORMANCE OBJECTIVE   The student will follow a routine procedure that meets the regulations and the protocol set forth by the dentist and regulatory agencies, keeping in mind that assistants' duties vary from state to state. The assistant may be evaluated by performance, statement, and/or combined responses and action. This procedure is performed by the dental assistant in the dental laboratory after the study model has set and been separated from the alginate impression and prepared for trimming.

	Self Evaluation	Student Evaluation	Possible Points	Instructor Evaluation	Comments
Equipment and Supplies					
1. Safety glasses			3		
2. Maxillary and mandibular models			3		
3. Two flexible rubber mixing bowls			3		
4. Laboratory knife			3		
5. Pencil			3		
6. Measuring straight edge			3		
Competency Steps					
1. Models need to be wet prior to trimming (if dry soak five minutes before trimming; trimming wheel on model trimmer works best with wet models).			3		
2. Put on safety glasses and adjust model trimmer (water to run freely over grinding wheel when trimmer turned on).			3		
3. Invert models so teeth are resting on counter. Evaluate whether base is parallel to counter. Art portion is one-half inch in when completed.			3		
4. Turn on model trimmer and trim base so it is parallel to occlusal plane. Hold model as level as possible (apply light, even pressure to models against grinding wheel on model trimmer).			3		
5. Rest hand on table of model trimmer. Keep fingers away from grinding wheel.			3		
6. Model may have to be returned to counter for re-evaluation and again to trimmer to achieve parallel surface. Trim both models to this stage.			3		
7. Place models together in occlusion (wax bite may be necessary), again re-evaluate. Models must be parallel. All other cuts will be off if this stage is not achieved.			3		

27-8 continued *(corresponds to textbook Procedure 27-12)*

	Self Evaluation	Student Evaluation	Possible Points	Instructor Evaluation	Comments
8. When cut maxillary and mandibular models as a pair are parallel, keep in occlusion and evaluate which posterior teeth are the most distal, maxillary or mandibular. Once determined, draw with the pencil a line behind the retromolar area indicating where to trim.			3		
9. Place base surface of model on model trimmer table guide and cut posterior area at right angle with base up to indicated lines.			3		
10. Put the two models back into occlusion and place cut model on top, whether it is maxillary or mandibular. Place opposite base on model trimmer table guide holding models together and trim posterior at a right angle to base (trimmed model will act as guide to follow while trimming).			3		
11. To evaluate, the models can be taken off the grinding wheel and placed on their backs. Occlusal plane is at right angle to counter. If models stay in occlusion, the objective has been met. If they fall apart, go back to grinding wheel until they stay.			3		
12. Trim heal, side, and anterior cuts:					
A. Mark outward from middle of mandibular premolars to edge of model			3		
B. Mark maxillary cuspids in same manner			3		
C. Draw line running parallel to teeth at greatest depth of buccal vestibule from molars to premolar			3		
D. Line will be about 5 mm from buccal surface of teeth			3		
E. Mark both sides of maxillary and mandibular model in this manner			3		
13. Place model base back on model trimmer table guide and trim model to pencil lines on both side. Repeat with both models.			3		
14. Mark with pencil a dot at midline of maxillary model in vestibule area. Using straight edge of measuring device, draw a line from dot to canine/cuspid line on each quadrant.			3		
15. Cut both anterior cuts, forming a pointed area at midline and center of both cuspids.			3		
16. After lines are drawn, make sure cuts will not trim away protruding teeth; if so, move lines out to accommodate. Model should appear symmetrical.			3		
17. The mandibular model is marked in rounded manner from middle of canine/cuspid on one side to middle of canine/cuspid on the other side. Pencil line can be drawn at depth of anterior vestibule as a guide for trimming.			3		

27-8 continued *(corresponds to textbook Procedure 27-12)*

	Self Evaluation	Student Evaluation	Possible Points	Instructor Evaluation	Comments
18. Heal cuts on both maxillary and mandibular models are three-eighths to five-eighths inches wide and should appear symmetric in length (can be drawn on model by turning base upward, placing imaginary diagonal line from cuspid (maxillary) premolar (mandibular) to where the side and back cuts meet; draw a 90° angle across base opposite anterior area; heal cuts are small on both maxillary and mandibular models that finish trimming of models).			3		
19. After models are trimmed symmetrically:					
A. With laboratory knife, trim tongue area flat and other art portion			3		
B. Any air bubbles fill with plaster			3		
C. Smooth flat surface with fine wet/dry sandpaper under water			3		
20. Models can be placed in a model gloss for ten minutes or sprayed with gloss for a professional appearance and to add strength (to achieve a high gloss, polish with dry cloth to buff).			3		
21. Final step is to label both models with patient's name, date model was taken. In an orthodontic office, patient's age may also be identified on model.			3		

TOTAL POINTS POSSIBLE   99

TOTAL POINTS POSSIBLE—2nd Attempt   97

TOTAL POINTS EARNED   _____

Points assigned reflect importance of step to meeting objective: Important = 1; Essential = 2; Critical = 3. Students will lose 2 points for repeated attempts. Failure results if any of the critical steps are omitted or performed incorrectly. If using a 100-point scale, determine score by dividing points earned by total points possible and multiplying the results by 100.

SCORE: _____

SKILL COMPETENCY ASSESSMENT

27-9 Constructing a Self-Cured Acrylic Resin Custom Tray
(corresponds to textbook Procedure 27-13)

Student's Name _____ Date _____

Instructor's Name _____

SKILL The dental assistant is responsible for preparation of equipment and supplies needed for appointments. The dentist may ask for a custom tray to be fabricated for the patient to obtain an accurate impression. This may be due to the fact that a regular stock tray does not fit. Several materials are available to make a custom tray. All materials used must be rigid enough to provide subsistence for the material as it is inserted and removed from the mouth. It is important that the material adapts well during the construction so that the final tray meets the required criteria.

PERFORMANCE OBJECTIVE The student will follow a routine procedure that meets the regulations and the protocol set forth by the dentist and regulatory agencies, keeping in mind that assistants' duties vary from state to state. The assistant may be evaluated by performance, statement, and/or combined responses and action. This procedure is performed by the dental assistant in the dental laboratory on a working cast.

	Self Evaluation	Student Evaluation	Possible Points	Instructor Evaluation	Comments
Equipment and Supplies					
1. Maxillary and/or mandibular casts			3		
2. Laboratory knife			3		
3. Pencil (plain or red and blue)			3		
4. Wax spatula			3		
5. Baseplate wax and heating source (warm water or laboratory torch)			3		
6. Tray resin with measuring devices			3		
7. Separating medium with brush			3		
8. Wooden tongue blade and wax-lined paper cup			3		
9. Petroleum jelly			3		
10. Tray adhesive			3		
Competency Steps					
Prepare the Cast					
1. Outline area of cast for spacer to be placed (2 to 3 mm below margin of prepared tooth or 2 to 3 mm above lowest point in vestibule if arch is edentulous).			3		
2. Fill any undercuts in cast. Heat spacer material and contour to the pencil line (undercuts can be covered with spacer material).			3		
3. Using laboratory knife, trim wax or spacer to line, using an angled cut instead of blunt cut.			3		
4. Cut appropriate stops in spacer.			3		
5. Cover spacer with aluminum foil or paint with separating medium.			3		

27-9 continued *(corresponds to textbook Procedure 27-13)*

	Self Evaluation	Student Evaluation	Possible Points	Instructor Evaluation	Comments
Mixing the Custom Tray Acrylic Self-Curing Resin					
1. Measure powder and liquid to correct calibrations on the measuring devices (follow manufacturer's directions).			3		
2. Mix powder and liquid together in wax-lined paper cup with wooden tongue blade until homogenous.			3		
3. Allow mixture to go through initial polymerization for 2 to 3 minutes (covering material during polymerization sometimes is indicated by manufacturer).			3		
4. During this time, place petroleum jelly over cast and palms of your hands.			3		
Contouring the Custom Tray Acrylic Self-Curing Resin					
1. When material is no longer sticky, gather into a ball, kneed material to further mix, and set small amount aside for handle.			3		
2. Place dough-like putty for maxillary cast					
A. Covering wax spacer			3		
B. Contour and adapt 1 to 2 mm over wax spacer			3		
C. Complete with rolled edge at designated area			3		
3. Adapt handle to custom tray (a drop of monomer liquid on tray where handle will be placed, will join better).			3		
4. Handle placed in midline area of the arch (if edentulous, handle should come up from ridge and then outward; with teeth, it can come directly outward).			3		
5. Handle should be placed and held in proper position until material becomes firm.			3		
Finishing the Custom Tray Acrylic Self-Curing Resin					
1. Setting will take about eight to ten minutes. Custom tray can be removed from cast and spacer material taken out.			3		
2. Clean tray			3		
A. If foil used, may take only a short time					
B. If wax, melt and remove using wax spatula, hot water, and toothbrush					
3. After final set, thirty minutes minimum, use acrylic bur or arbor band to trim edges of tray (do not trim inside).			3		
4. Clean and disinfect tray, write patient's name on tray (disinfect following manufacturer's directions).			3		

27-9 **continued** *(corresponds to textbook Procedure 27-13)*

	Self Evaluation	Student Evaluation	Possible Points	Instructor Evaluation	Comments
5. Apply adhesive to inside of tray and along margins (adhesive provided by manufacturer).			3		

TOTAL POINTS POSSIBLE   93

TOTAL POINTS POSSIBLE—2nd Attempt   91

TOTAL POINTS EARNED   _____

Points assigned reflect importance of step to meeting objective: Important = 1; Essential = 2; Critical = 3. Students will lose 2 points for repeated attempts. Failure results if any of the critical steps are omitted or performed incorrectly. If using a 100-point scale, determine score by dividing points earned by total points possible and multiplying the results by 100.

SCORE: _____

SKILL COMPETENCY ASSESSMENT

27-10 Constructing a Vacuum-Formed Acrylic Resin Custom Tray
(corresponds to textbook Procedure 27-14)

Student's Name _____ Date _____

Instructor's Name _____

SKILL   The dental assistant is responsible for preparation of equipment and supplies needed for appointments. The dentist may ask for a custom tray to be fabricated for the patient to obtain an accurate impression. This may be due to the fact that a regular stock tray does not fit. Several materials are available to make a custom tray. All materials used must be rigid enough to provide subsistence for the material as it is inserted and removed from the mouth. It is important that the material adapts well during the construction so that the final tray meets the required criteria. The vacuum-formed custom trays require additional equipment. This unit has a frame that holds a sheet directly under a heating element and when the sheet is softened, the frame drops the sheet onto the cast as a vacuum pressure draws the material to the model.

PERFORMANCE OBJECTIVE   The student will follow a routine procedure that meets the regulations and the protocol set forth by the dentist and regulatory agencies, keeping in mind that assistants' duties vary from state to state. The assistant may be evaluated by performance, statement, and/or combined responses and action. This procedure is performed by the dental assistant in the dental laboratory on a working cast.

	Self Evaluation	Student Evaluation	Possible Points	Instructor Evaluation	Comments
Equipment and Supplies					
1. Maxillary and/or mandibular cast			3		
2. Laboratory knife			3		
3. Laboratory scissors			3		
4. Vacuum former with heating element			3		
5. Acrylic sheets			3		
Competency Steps					
Preparing the Cast					
1. Soaking cast recommended prior to forming custom tray on it (up to thirty minutes prior— eliminates air bubbles during heating phase).			3		
2. Place spacer if indicated (wax spacer will melt under heat).			3		
3. Mark desired outer margin of custom tray to be made.			3		
4. Place cast on platform of vacuum-forming unit.			3		
Contouring the Acrylic Resin Sheets during the Vacuum-Forming Process					
1. Select appropriate acrylic resin sheet used for the product.			3		
2. Acrylic resin sheets placed between heater frame and gasket frame, anterior knob tight to secure material in place.			3		
3. Heating element must be in correct place, (above acrylic resin sheet). Turn it on.			3		
4. As resin heats, it will begin to sag downward. Allow to droop down to about one inch (over- heating causes air bubbles to form on surface of acrylic resin).			3		

27-10 continued *(corresponds to textbook Procedure 27-14)*

	Self Evaluation	Student Evaluation	Possible Points	Instructor Evaluation	Comments
5. After material heated properly, take both handles on frame and pull downward over cast (only touch handles as entire area is extremely hot).			3		
6. Turn on vacuum immediately after resin sheet is entirely over the cast.			3		
7. Turn off heating unit.			3		
8. Allow vacuum to continue for one to two minutes (resin to cool and become firm again).			3		
Finishing the Vacuum-Formed Acrylic Resin Custom Tray					
1. After resin material cooled, remove from vacuum form frame.			3		
2. Separate resin-formed custom tray from cast and trim to desired form with laboratory scissors.			3		
3. Prepare cutout handle section to custom tray (using torch as heat).			3		
4. Clean and disinfect custom tray according to manufacturer's directions. Write patient's name on it.			3		

TOTAL POINTS POSSIBLE   63

TOTAL POINTS POSSIBLE—2nd Attempt   61

TOTAL POINTS EARNED   _____

Points assigned reflect importance of step to meeting objective: Important = 1; Essential = 2; Critical = 3. Students will lose 2 points for repeated attempts. Failure results if any of the critical steps are omitted or performed incorrectly. If using a 100-point scale, determine score by dividing points earned by total points possible and multiplying the results by 100.

SCORE: _____

SKILL COMPETENCY ASSESSMENT

27-11 Sizing, Adapting, and Seating a Preformed Acrylic Crown
(corresponds to textbook Procedure 27-17)

Student's Name _____ Date _____

Instructor's Name _____

SKILL The dental assistant is responsible for preparation of equipment and supplies needed for appointments. After a tooth has been prepared for a crown and prior to the seating of the crown, a temporary restoration must be adapted and temporary cemented on the tooth to protect it in the interim time. These temporary restorations stabilize and protect the tooth for the period it takes to make the crown(s) or bridge(s). Temporary restorations also known as provisional restorations can be made of a number of materials. Preformed acrylic or plastic temporary crowns are available in different sizes, shapes, and shades. The advantage to this crown is that it is more esthetically pleasing for anterior use. The preformed acrylic crowns are more easily used because they have little adjustment and can be immediately seated.

PERFORMANCE OBJECTIVE The student will follow a routine procedure that meets the regulations and the protocol set forth by the dentist and regulatory agencies, keeping in mind that assistants' duties vary from state to state. The assistant may be evaluated by performance, statement, and/or combined responses and action. This procedure is performed by the dentist or the dental assistant at the dental unit after the preformed acrylic provisional has been prepared and sized and contoured to the prepared tooth.

	Self Evaluation	Student Evaluation	Possible Points	Instructor Evaluation	Comments
Equipment and Supplies					
1. Maxillary and/or mandibular selection of acrylic temporary crowns			3		
2. Basic setup: mouth mirror, explorer, cotton pliers			3		
3. Acrylic or composite temporary material (optional)			3		
4. Acrylic bur			3		
5. Temporary cement, pad, and spatula			3		
6. Articulating paper			3		
7. Dental floss			3		
Competency Steps					
Preparing the Preformed Acrylic Temporary Restoration					
1. After tooth prepared for crown, a preformed acrylic temporary can be selected and adapted.			3		
2. Crown chosen for proper tooth			3		
A. Wide enough to contact adjacent teeth			3		
B. Long enough for proper occlusion			3		
C. Correct shade			3		
3. Retrieve crown without cross-contaminating other acrylic crowns (tab on incisal edge allows operator to try crown over prepared tooth).			3		
4. Adjustments made with acrylic bur, polished with rag wheel and pumice (adjustments as needed for fit).			3		
5. Take off tag, place crown in place, and check occlusion with articulating paper.			3		

27-11 continued *(corresponds to textbook Procedure 27-17)*

	Self Evaluation	Student Evaluation	Possible Points	Instructor Evaluation	Comments
6. If further adjustments are necessary, do so. Again polish adjustment areas for a smooth surface for patient comfort.			3		
Cementing the Acrylic Provisional Crown					
1. Rinse and dry prepared tooth with cotton rolls in place.			3		
2. Temporary cementation material mixed with spatula, placed into preformed acrylic crown.			3		
3. Preformed acrylic crown is placed into position, over prepared tooth. Patient is asked to bite in occlusion until cement is set (or operator will hold it in place).			3		
4. After cement is set, excess is removed with explorer.			3		
5. Contacts are checked with floss			3		
A. Margins are all inspected to see whether all excess cement was removed			3		
B. Crown fits correctly			3		
6. Final check for occlusion is done with articulating paper.			3		
7. Instructions are given to patient for care of temporary preformed acrylic crown.			3		

TOTAL POINTS POSSIBLE   75

TOTAL POINTS POSSIBLE—2nd Attempt   73

TOTAL POINTS EARNED   _____

Points assigned reflect importance of step to meeting objective: Important = 1; Essential = 2; Critical = 3. Students will lose 2 points for repeated attempts. Failure results if any of the critical steps are omitted or performed incorrectly. If using a 100-point scale, determine score by dividing points earned by total points possible and multiplying the results by 100.

SCORE: _____

SKILL COMPETENCY ASSESSMENT

27-12 Adapting, Trimming, and Seating a Matrix and Custom Temporary Restoration *(corresponds to textbook Procedure 27-18)*

Student's Name _____ Date _____

Instructor's Name _____

SKILL   The dental assistant is responsible for preparation of equipment and supplies needed for appointments. After a tooth has been prepared for a crown and prior to the seating of the crown, a temporary restoration must be adapted and temporary cemented on the tooth to protect it in the interim time. These temporary restorations stabilize and protect the tooth for the period it takes to make the crown(s) or bridge(s). Temporary restorations also known as provisional restorations can be made of a number of materials. In making custom acrylic or composite temporary restorations, a matrix is used. A custom acrylic or composite temporary restoration must have good proximal contacts, good occlusal contacts, good food deflection, and good marginal contours.

PERFORMANCE OBJECTIVE   The student will follow a routine procedure that meets the regulations and the protocol set forth by the dentist and regulatory agencies, keeping in mind that assistants' duties vary from state to state. The assistant may be evaluated by performance, statement, and/or combined responses and action. This procedure is performed by the dentist or the dental assistant at the dental unit after the tooth has been prepared for a crown.

	Self Evaluation	Student Evaluation	Possible Points	Instructor Evaluation	Comments
Equipment and Supplies					
1. Basic setup: mouth mirror, explorer, cotton pliers			3		
2. Thermo-plastic buttons/hot water (one option to make matrix)			3		
3. Composite temporary material			3		
4. Diamond bur			3		
5. Temporary cement, pad, and spatula			3		
6. Articulating paper			3		
7. Dental floss			3		
Competency Steps					
Making the Thermo-Forming Matrix Prior to the Tooth Preparation					
1. Place thermo-forming matrix buttons in hot water (one per tooth).			3		
2. Allow white color of button to become clear (indicates material is pliable and able to be adapted).			3		
3. Adapt material over tooth to be prepared and tightly conform it to tooth area and slightly below gingival.			3		
4. When material cools, matrix will appear white and firm (air can be used to make this more rapid).			3		
5. Remove matrix from area and set aside.			3		
Preparing the Custom Temporary Restoration					
1. After tooth has been prepared for crown, coat teeth with light application of petroleum jelly.			3		
2. Dispense self-curing material onto paper pad by holding tubes at 45° angle (this applies to					

27-12 continued *(corresponds to textbook Procedure 27-18)*

	Self Evaluation	Student Evaluation	Possible Points	Instructor Evaluation	Comments
composite self-curing temporary material in two tubes).			3		
3. Method of dispensing:					
A. Larger of two tubes is base—rotate end-dispensing handle until a click is heard			3		
B. Smaller of the two holds catalyst and has two dispensing ends—rotate end-dispensing handle and two small amounts will be expelled			3		
C. Dispense both tubes (one tube has two small tips that will each click enough material for one temporary)			3		
4. If shade is being used, mix with base prior to bringing materials together (mottled effect desired, mix shade after base and catalyst are mixed together).			3		
5. Mix material together to obtain a creamy substance (thirty seconds).			3		
6. Place material into matrix.			3		
7. Place matrix over prepared tooth (manipulation time one and one-half minutes).			3		
8. Hold in place for two minutes in mouth.			3		
9. Remove from mouth and set aside for two minutes.			3		
10. Remove from matrix.			3		
11. Additional curing time will take one minute.			3		
12. Seven minutes total time from start to finish of set.			3		
13. Remove greasy layer with alcohol or any other solvent.			3		
14. Trim with a diamond or acrylic bur.			3		
15. Check contacts with floss.			3		
16. Check occlusion with articulating paper and having patient bite.			3		
17. Check margins with explorer and mirror.			3		

TOTAL POINTS POSSIBLE   93

TOTAL POINTS POSSIBLE—2nd Attempt   91

TOTAL POINTS EARNED   _____

Points assigned reflect importance of step to meeting objective: Important = 1; Essential = 2; Critical = 3. Students will lose 2 points for repeated attempts. Failure results if any of the critical steps are omitted or performed incorrectly. If using a 100-point scale, determine score by dividing points earned by total points possible and multiplying the results by 100.

SCORE: _____

SKILL COMPETENCY ASSESSMENT

27-13 Cementing the Custom Self-Curing Composite Temporary Crown
(corresponds to textbook Procedure 27-19)

Student's Name _____ Date _____

Instructor's Name _____

SKILL   The dental assistant is responsible for preparation of equipment and supplies needed for appointments. After a tooth has been prepared for a crown and prior to the seating of the crown, a temporary restoration must be adapted and temporary cemented on the tooth to protect it in the interim time. These temporary restorations stabilize and protect the tooth for the period it takes to make the crown(s) or bridge(s). Temporary restorations also known as provisional restorations can be made of a number of materials.

PERFORMANCE OBJECTIVE   The student will follow a routine procedure that meets the regulations and the protocol set forth by the dentist and regulatory agencies, keeping in mind that assistants' duties vary from state to state. The assistant may be evaluated by performance, statement, and/or combined responses and action. This procedure is performed by the dentist or the dental assistant at the dental unit after the tooth temporary restoration has been prepared and is ready to be cemented.

	Self Evaluation	Student Evaluation	Possible Points	Instructor Evaluation	Comments
Equipment and Supplies					
1. Basic setup: mouth mirror, explorer, cotton pliers			3		
2. Cotton rolls			3		
3. Temporary luting cement			3		
4. Paper pad			3		
5. Mixing spatula			3		
6. Plastic filling instrument			3		
7. Dental floss			3		
Competency Steps					
1. Prepared tooth rinsed and dried with cotton rolls in place.			3		
2. Temporary cement material mixed with spatula and placed into custom composite temporary crown.			3		
3. Temporary crown placed in position over prepared tooth. Patient asked to bite in occlusion until cement set.			3		
4. After cement is set, excess is removed with an explorer.			3		
5. Contacts checked with floss, margins inspected, determine all excess cement has been removed, crown fits correctly.			3		
6. Final check for occlusion done with articulating paper.			3		

27-13 continued *(corresponds to textbook Procedure 27-19)*

	Self Evaluation	Student Evaluation	Possible Points	Instructor Evaluation	Comments
7. Instructions are given to patient for care of custom composite temporary crown.			3		

TOTAL POINTS POSSIBLE	42	
TOTAL POINTS POSSIBLE—2nd Attempt	40	
TOTAL POINTS EARNED	_____	

Points assigned reflect importance of step to meeting objective: Important = 1; Essential = 2; Critical = 3. Students will lose 2 points for repeated attempts. Failure results if any of the critical steps are omitted or performed incorrectly. If using a 100-point scale, determine score by dividing points earned by total points possible and multiplying the results by 100.

SCORE: _____

Advanced Chairside Functions

OBJECTIVES

Refer to textbook pages 627 through 686 for individual Objective Lists for the following expanded functions: Dental Dam; Matrix and Wedge; Coronal Polish; Placing Cavity Liners, Cavity Varnish, and Cement Bases; Suture Removal; Gingival Retraction; and Bleaching Techniques.

SUMMARY

Expanded functions, such as dental dam placement, matrix and wedge placement and removal, performance of a coronal polish, cavity preparation, suture removal, gingival retraction, application of enamel sealants, and bleaching, are specific advanced tasks that require increased skill and responsibility. These functions are delegated by the dentist according to the Dental Practice Act within the state. Some states require additional education, certification, or registration to perform these functions.

KEY TERMS

anchor tooth
cervical clamps
dental dam clamps
dental dam forceps
dental dam frame

dental dam napkins
dental dam punch
interseptal
inverting
key hole punch

ligature
septum
template
winged clamps
wingless clamps

EXERCISES AND ACTIVITIES

Dental Dam

1. The dental dam procedure requires a variety of instruments and materials. The most common adult size of precut rubber dam material is _____
   - A. 5 x 5
   - B. 6 x 6
   - C. 5 x 6
   - D. 6 x 5

2. What dental dam instrument has a working end that is a sharp projection used to provide holes in the dam? _____
   - A. Clamp
   - B. Punch
   - C. Forceps
   - D. Pliers

3. Dental dam clamps are designed to be used on specific teeth. One of the basic parts of the clamp is the arched metal joining the two jaws of the clamp together, called the _____
   - A. points.
   - B. wings.
   - C. bow.
   - D. hole.

4. Scissors are used to cut the _____ dental dam during removal of the dam from the patient's mouth.
   - A. stabilizing cord
   - B. interseptal
   - C. face napkin
   - D. floss

5. There are many advantages to using the dental dam; however, there are conditions that contraindicate the use of the dental dam. Which of the following are contraindications? _____
   1. Provides greater visibility
   2. Latex allergies
   3. Respiratory congestion
   4. Herpetic lesions
   5. Retracts tongue
   6. Provides greater accessibility

   - A. 1, 2, 5
   - B. 2, 3, 6
   - C. 2, 3, 4
   - D. 1, 3, 5

Matrix and Wedge

6. The most commonly used matrix in an amalgam restoration is the _____
   - A. strip.
   - B. shell.
   - C. Tofflemire.
   - D. AutoMatrix.

7. Which matrix is used without a retainer for an amalgam restoration? _____
   - A. Strip
   - B. Shell
   - C. Tofflemire
   - D. AutoMatrix

8. Which part of the Tofflemire matrix retainer holds the ends of the matrix band in place in the diagonal slot? _____
   - A. Spindle
   - B. Vise
   - C. Guide channels
   - D. Inner knob

9. After the Tofflemire matrix is assembled and positioned on the tooth, the band of the matrix should extend no more than _____ beyond the gingival margin.
   - A. 2.0 mm
   - B. 1.0 mm
   - C. 1.75 mm
   - D. 3.0 mm

Coronal Polish

10. _____ stains are found inside the tooth structure and are mostly permanent.
    - A. Intrinsic
    - B. Extrinsic
    - C. Endogenous
    - D. Tobacco

11. Which of the following is not an extrinsic stain? _____
    - A. Yellow
    - B. Green
    - C. Dark grey-brown
    - D. Black

12. There are many benefits and indications for a coronal polish. Which of the following are not? _____
    1. Could traumatize tissues
    2. Easier to keep teeth clean
    3. Tooth surface absorbs fluoride better
    4. Could cause gingival irritation
    5. Gingival tissues hemorrhage easily
    6. Motivates patient to maintain good oral hygiene

    - A. 1, 4, 5
    - B. 1, 3, 4
    - C. 2, 3, 4
    - D. 2, 3, 6

Placing Cement Bases, Cavity Liners, and Cavity Varnish

13. An ideal cavity preparation would suggest what type of treatment as related to pulpal involvement? _____
    - A. Direct pulp capping
    - B. Two thin layers of liner
    - C. Cavity varnish
    - D. No treatment required prior to restoration

14. A cement base is mixed to what consistency? _____
    A. Putty   C. Flowing
    B. Luting   D. Powder

Suture Removal

15. Prior to suture removal, several steps and considerations are necessary to ensure patient comfort and safety. Which of the following is not a consideration? _____
    A. Examine suture site
    B. Review patient's chart
    C. Evaluate appearance of suture site
    D. Review patient's payment program

16. There are various types of suture patterns. The most widely used and versatile stitch is the _____
    A. sling.   C. continuous.
    B. simple.   D. mattress.

17. When a flap has been necessary, which type of suture is especially useful? _____
    A. Sling   C. Continuous
    B. Simple   D. Mattress

Gingival Retraction

18. Which of the following is not a form of gingival retraction? _____
    A. Chemical   C. Mechanical
    B. Cotton roll   D. Surgical

Enamel Sealants

19. The enamel surface is "etched" in preparation for sealants. What is the etchant application time? _____
    A. Thirty to sixty seconds
    B. Thirty to ninety seconds
    C. Five minutes
    D. Twenty to thirty seconds

20. This type of sealant material is known as self-cure or autopolymerization. _____
    A. Light cured   B. Chemically cured

21. Enamel sealants are most beneficial if indicated. Which of the following would be indications to placing enamel sealants? _____
    1. Caries within the past two years
    2. Teeth with shallow open grooves
    3. Teeth recently erupted
    4. Occlusal pits and fissures on non-carious primary and permanent teeth
    5. Teeth with occlusal restorations
    6. Along with preventive treatment

    A. 1, 2, 6
    B. 2, 3, 5
    C. 3, 4, 6
    D. 1, 4, 6

Bleaching

22. Which type of bleaching is used to lighten an endodontically treated tooth? _____
    A. Non-vital
    B. Dental office
    C. At home
    D. Vital

23. Power bleaching is accomplished on _____ teeth.
    A. non-vital
    B. vital
    C. endodontic
    D. None of the above

24. Which of the following is not among the most commonly used bleaching agents? _____
    A. Sodium perborate
    B. Sodium bicarbonate
    C. Hydrogen peroxide
    D. Carbamide peroxide

SKILL COMPETENCY ASSESSMENT

│28-1 Placing and Removing the Dental Dam

Student's Name _____ Date _____

Instructor's Name _____

SKILL Routine steps should be followed for all treatment areas to maintain absolute clinical asepsis. The dental assistant is responsible for preparation of equipment and supplies needed for appointments. There are many techniques for placement of the dental dam and the operator will find through practice what works best.

PERFORMANCE OBJECTIVE The student will follow a routine procedure that meets the regulations and the protocol set forth by the dentist and regulatory agencies, keeping in mind that assistants' duties vary from state to state. The assistant may be evaluated by performance, statement, and/or combined responses and action. This procedure is performed by the dentist or the dental assistant. The patient has been anesthetized before the placement of the dental dam and before the cavity preparation begins. Only the items for the dental dam will be listed for this procedure.

	Self Evaluation	Student Evaluation	Possible Points	Instructor Evaluation	Comments
Equipment and Supplies					
1. Dental dam material (6 x 6 sheets)			3		
2. Dental dam napkin			3		
3. Dental dam punch			3		
4. Assortment of clamps			3		
5. Dental dam forceps			3		
6. Dental dam frame			3		
7. Dental floss			3		
8. Lubricant			3		
9. Cotton-tip applicator			3		
10. Tucking instrument			3		
11. Scissors			3		
Competency Steps					
Placement of the Dental Dam					
1. Inform patient on dental dam procedure.			3		
2. Examine patient's oral cavity to determine:					
A. Anchor tooth			3		
B. Shape of arch			3		
C. Tooth alignment			3		
D. Missing teeth			3		
E. Presence of crowns or bridges			3		
F. Gingival tissue condition			2		
G. Tight contacts			3		
3. Prepare dam material by dividing it into sixths, and punch dam, aligning stylus and holes carefully.			3		
4. Center the punch in upper or lower middle third of dam.			3		

28-1 continued

	Self Evaluation	Student Evaluation	Possible Points	Instructor Evaluation	Comments
5. Holes punched according to size of tooth, key punch being largest to accommodate anchor tooth and clamp.			3		
6. Holes punched following pattern of patient's arch. Lubricate dental dam on tissue side of dam (water-soluble lubricant).			3		
7. Select clamp or several clamps to try on tooth (selection: design—winged/wingless; mesiodistal width, faciolingual width—both at CEJ of anchor tooth; height of occlusal plane of anchor tooth).			3		
8. Attach safety line on all clamps to be tried on.			3		
9. Secure clamp on forceps and spread jaws slightly to lock forceps.			3		
10. Place clamp over anchor tooth (to widen jaws, squeeze forceps handle slightly to release locking bar).			3		
11. Fitting jaws of clamp:					
A. Fit lingual jaw of clamp on lingual side of tooth first			3		
B. Next spread clamp and slide buccal jaws of clamp over height of contour of buccal surface of tooth			3		
C. Release pressure on clamp forceps slightly against tooth to evaluate clamp, but do not release clamp from forceps			3		
12. Clamp on tooth:					
A. Jaw points at CEJ			3		
B. Jaws adapting to gingival embrasures on the buccal and lingual			3		
C. Clamp secure			3		
D. Not pinching any gingival tissue			3		
E. Confirm with patient about comfort			3		
13. Place dental dam over clamp bow:					
A. Grasp dam material with index fingers on each side of key punch hole			3		
B. Spread hole wide enough to slip over clamp			3		
C. Stretch hole over anchor tooth and one side of clamp			3		
D. Expose other clamp jaw—entire clamp and tooth exposed			3		
E. Pull safety line through dam and drape to side of patient's mouth			3		
14. Isolate most forward tooth, usually opposite canine, dam material secured on distal of tooth (with double loop of floss, a corner cut of dam or stabilizing cord).			3		
15. Place dental napkin around patient's mouth.			3		

28-1 continued

	Self Evaluation	Student Evaluation	Possible Points	Instructor Evaluation	Comments
16. Place frame or holder to stretch dam to cover oral cavity (frame can be placed either under or over dental dam material depending on type of frame and preference of operator).			3		
17. Isolate remaining teeth:					
A. Dental dam worked gently between contacts			3		
B. Dental floss used to assist placing dam and exposing teeth			3		
C. Use air syringe to dry teeth			3		
18. Invert or tuck dam material (edge of dam that surrounds tooth must be inverted or tucked into sulcus of gingiva to seal tooth and prevent leakage).			3		
19. Coat all tooth-colored restorations with lubricant.			3		
20. Place and position saliva ejector and/or bite block under dam for patient comfort as needed.			3		
21. Double-check dam placement and patient comfort.			3		
Removal of the Dental Dam *When the operator is ready to remove the dental dam, the area is rinsed and dried using the evacuator and the three-way syringe.*					
1. Explain to patient procedure to remove dental dam; caution them not to bite down during removal.			3		
2. Free interseptal dam with scissors, protect patient's lip, scissors to clip each septum.			3		
3. Remove dental dam clamp (lift straight off tooth).			3		
4. Remove frame or holder of dam material.			3		
5. Remove napkin, wiping area around mouth.			3		
6. Examine dam material, spreading material out flat to make certain all interseptal material is present (any missing pieces, floss between teeth and dislodge remaining dam).			3		
7. Massage gingiva around anchor tooth.			3		
8. Rinse patient's mouth thoroughly.			3		
TOTAL POINTS POSSIBLE			173		
TOTAL POINTS POSSIBLE—2nd Attempt			171		
TOTAL POINTS EARNED			_____		

Points assigned reflect importance of step to meeting objective: Important = 1; Essential = 2; Critical = 3. Students will lose 2 points for repeated attempts. Failure results if any of the critical steps are omitted or performed incorrectly. If using a 100-point scale, determine score by dividing points earned by total points possible and multiplying the results by 100.

SCORE: _____

SKILL COMPETENCY ASSESSMENT

28-2 Assembly of the Tofflemire Matrix *(corresponds to textbook Procedure 28-4)*

Student's Name _____ Date _____

Instructor's Name _____

SKILL Routine steps should be followed for all treatment areas to maintain absolute clinical asepsis. The dental assistant is responsible for preparation of equipment and supplies needed for the appointment. During the preparation of a tooth for an amalgam or a composite restoration, often one or more axial surfaces will be removed. A matrix replaces the surface and acts as the artificial wall. The Tofflemire matrix is the most common matrix used for amalgam restorations. It has two parts: the retainer and the band.

PERFORMANCE OBJECTIVE The student will follow a routine procedure that meets the regulations and the protocol set forth by the dentist and regulatory agencies, keeping in mind that assistants' duties vary from state to state. The assistant may be evaluated by performance, statement, and/or combined responses and action. This procedure is performed by the dentist or the dental assistant. The assembly can be completed before the procedure begins so it is ready when needed. Equipment and supplies listed are for the assembly of the Tofflemire matrix.

	Self Evaluation	Student Evaluation	Possible Points	Instructor Evaluation	Comments
Equipment and Supplies					
1. Tofflemire retainer			3		
2. Assortment of matrix bands			3		
Competency Steps					
1. Hold retainer so guide channels and diagonal slot on vise are facing operator.			3		
2. Holding frame of retainer, rotate inner knob until vise is within one-quarter inch of guide channels.			3		
3. Turn outer knob until pointed end of spindle is clear of slot in vise.			3		
4. Prepare matrix band for placement in retainer, holding band (like smile), gingival edge on top, occlusal edge on bottom.			3		
5. Bring ends together to form a teardrop-shaped loop (do not crease; larger circumference of band, occlusal, on bottom and smaller, gingival, on top).			3		
6. Gingival edge still on top, place occlusal edge of band into diagonal slot of vise. Loop will extend toward guide channels.			3		
7. Place matrix band into appropriate guide channels. Direction of matrix band depends on tooth being restored.			3		
Hold matrix retainer with guide channel up, facing operator, and the matrix band looped. Then:					
A. Maxillary right/mandibular left quadrant, matrix will be placed in guide channels toward operator's right			3		

28-2 continued *(corresponds to textbook Procedure 28-4)*

	Self Evaluation	Student Evaluation	Possible Points	Instructor Evaluation	Comments
B. Maxillary left/mandibular right quadrant, matrix will be placed in guide channels toward operator's left			3		
8. Once band is placed in slot with guide channels, turn outer knob until tip of spindle is tight against band in vise slot.			3		
9. Move inner knob to increase or decrease the size of loop to match diameter of tooth.			3		
10. Smooth out band—eliminate creasing, (handle of mouth mirror, similar to curling ribbon).			3		

TOTAL POINTS POSSIBLE   42

TOTAL POINTS POSSIBLE—2nd Attempt   40

TOTAL POINTS EARNED   _____

Points assigned reflect importance of step to meeting objective: Important = 1; Essential = 2; Critical = 3. Students will lose 2 points for repeated attempts. Failure results if any of the critical steps are omitted or performed incorrectly. If using a 100-point scale, determine score by dividing points earned by total points possible and multiplying the results by 100.

SCORE: _____

SKILL COMPETENCY ASSESSMENT

28-3 Coronal Polish *(corresponds to textbook Procedure 28-12)*

Student's Name _____ Date _____

Instructor's Name _____

SKILL   Routine steps should be followed for all treatment areas to maintain absolute clinical asepsis. The dental assistant is responsible for preparation of equipment and supplies needed for the appointment. The coronal polish procedure involves removing soft deposits and extrinsic stains from the surfaces of the teeth and restorations. This is accomplished with an abrasive, dental handpiece, a rubber cup, a brush, dental tape and floss. It is helpful to follow a systematic procedure when polishing the entire mouth by developing a sequence that is always followed.

PERFORMANCE OBJECTIVE   The student will follow a routine procedure that meets the regulations and the protocol set forth by the dentist and regulatory agencies, keeping in mind that assistants' duties vary from state to state. The assistant may be evaluated by performance, statement and/or combined responses and action. This procedure is performed by the dental assistant and the dental hygienist. This procedure describes the protocol for performing a coronal polish including preparation of materials, the patient, positioning of the operator and the patient, sequence of procedure, and evaluating the procedure. The details of use of the rubber cup, brush, and dental tape and floss have been described previously in this section.

	Self Evaluation	Student Evaluation	Possible Points	Instructor Evaluation	Comments
Equipment and Supplies					
1. Basic setup: mouth mirror, explorer, cotton pliers			3		
2. Saliva ejector, HVE tip, air-water syringe tip			3		
3. 2 x 2 gauze sponges, cotton-tip applicators, tongue blade, and cotton rolls			3		
4. Lip lubricant and disclosing solution in dappen dish			3		
5. Low-speed handpiece with prophy angle attachment			3		
6. Prophy cups and brushes (dappen dish with warm water to soak brushes in)			3		
7. Prophy pastes, with a variety of grits and finger ring holder			3		
8. Dental tape and dental floss			3		
9. Auxiliary aids as needed			3		
The following items are needed off the tray:					
1. Patient's chart			3		
2. Red/blue pencil, lead pencil, and pen			3		
3. Barriers for the dental unit			3		
4. Patient napkin and napkin chain			3		
5. Patient safety glasses			3		
6. Patient hand mirror			3		
Competency Steps					
1. Gather above equipment and materials, prepare operatory for patient, review patient's records.			3		

28-3 continued *(corresponds to textbook Procedure 28-12)*

	Self Evaluation	Student Evaluation	Possible Points	Instructor Evaluation	Comments
2. Prepare the patient:					
A. Follow established procedure, seat patient, review/update patient's records			3		
B. Explain procedure to patient			3		
C. Follow aseptic procedures, prepare patient for coronal polish			3		
D. Evaluate patient's condition, perform oral inspection			3		
E. Select abrasive agents to be used after examining teeth			3		
F. Lubricate patient's lips, dry teeth, apply closing agent with cotton-tip applicator			3		
G. Adjust dental unit light for good vision			3		
3. Positioning of the operator and the patient:					
A. Demonstrate position of operator and patient			3		
B. Demonstrate position of patient's head 1. Turned away from operator when operator polishing maxillary/mandibular right facial and maxillary/mandibular left lingual			3		
2. Turned toward operator when operator polishing maxillary/mandibular right lingual and maxillary/mandibular left facial			3		
4. Sequence of procedure:					
A. Begin polish on quadrant you decided would be beginning point			3		
B. Follow criteria previously on use of abrasives, rubber cup, prophy brush, tape, and floss			3		
C. Rinse patient's mouth after each quadrant, or as needed for comfort			3		
5. Evaluating the coronal polish:					
A. Once all steps of coronal polish are complete, rinse patient's mouth thoroughly with spray from air-water syringe and evacuate			3		
B. Apply disclosing solution to detect any areas of plaque or stain missed			3		
C. Using mouth mirror and air syringe, inspect each surface for any remaining soft deposits and/or stains			3		
D. Note these areas on chart for future reference			3		
E. Polish areas missed with prophy cup and/or brush			3		
F. Rinse patient's mouth to remove all abrasive agent			3		
G. Inspect teeth for lustrous shine with no debris or extrinsic stains; soft tissues should be free of abrasion or trauma			3		
H. The patient is ready for fluoride treatments			3		
I. The dentist may want to see patient before patient is dismissed			3		

28-3 continued *(corresponds to textbook Procedure 28-12)*

	Self Evaluation	Student Evaluation	Possible Points	Instructor Evaluation	Comments
6. Charting the coronal polish:					
A. Assistant's responsibility to record coronal polish completely and accurately on patient's dental chart			3		
B. Entry is recorded in ink, dated, signed, or entered into computer system			3		
C. Include any comments about condition of patient's mouth and type(s) of material(s) used			3		
TOTAL POINTS POSSIBLE			126		
TOTAL POINTS POSSIBLE—2nd Attempt			124		
TOTAL POINTS EARNED			_____		

Points assigned reflect importance of step to meeting objective: Important = 1; Essential = 2; Critical = 3. Students will lose 2 points for repeated attempts. Failure results if any of the critical steps are omitted or performed incorrectly. If using a 100-point scale, determine score by dividing points earned by total points possible and multiplying the results by 100.

SCORE: _____

SKILL COMPETENCY ASSESSMENT

28-4 Placing Cavity Liners *(corresponds to textbook Procedure 28-13)*

Student's Name _____ Date _____

Instructor's Name _____

SKILL Routine steps should be followed for all treatment areas to maintain absolute clinical asepsis. The dental assistant is responsible for preparation of equipment and supplies needed for the appointment. Dental liners are placed in the deepest portion of the cavity preparation on the axial or pulpal walls. After the liners are hardened, they form a cement layer with minimum strength.

PERFORMANCE OBJECTIVE The student will follow a routine procedure that meets the regulations and the protocol set forth by the dentist and regulatory agencies, keeping in mind that assistants' duties vary from state to state. The assistant may be evaluated by performance, statement, and/or combined responses and action. This procedure is performed by the dentist or an expanded-functions dental assistant. The preparation of the cavity has been completed, and this procedure begins the restorative process.

	Self Evaluation	Student Evaluation	Possible Points	Instructor Evaluation	Comments
Equipment and Supplies					
1. Cavity liner (calcium hydroxide, glass ionomer, zinc oxide eugenol)			3		
2. Application instrument—small, balled instrument or explorer			3		
3. Gauze sponges and cotton rolls			3		
4. Mixing pad and spatula, if material is needed			3		
5. Curing light (if material is light cured)			3		
Competency Steps					
1. Examine cavity preparation. Determine deepest portion of cavity preparation and access to that area.			3		
2. Clean and dry cavity preparation, remove any debris from cavity preparation, wash and dry area with air-water syringe.			3		
3. Prepare liner to be used. Dispense and mix according to directions.			3		
4. Place liner in cavity preparation. Using small, ball-ended instrument, place material in deepest portion of cavity preparation in a thin layer.			3		
5. Complete the placement, remove instrument, wipe it clean with gauze, and repeat procedure until liner covers deepest portion of cavity preparation.			3		
6. Light curing of liner:					
A. If liner is self-curing, the mix must be allowed to harden			3		
B. If liner is light curing, light is held over tooth and activated to cure for appropriate time (usually ten to twenty seconds)			3		

28-4 continued *(corresponds to textbook Procedure 28-13)*

	Self Evaluation	Student Evaluation	Possible Points	Instructor Evaluation	Comments
7. Examine cavity preparation. After liner has cured, examine preparation. If any material is on enamel walls, remove with explorer.			3		

TOTAL POINTS POSSIBLE	39	
TOTAL POINTS POSSIBLE—2nd Attempt	37	
TOTAL POINTS EARNED	_____	

Points assigned reflect importance of step to meeting objective: Important = 1; Essential = 2; Critical = 3. Students will lose 2 points for repeated attempts. Failure results if any of the critical steps are omitted or performed incorrectly. If using a 100-point scale, determine score by dividing points earned by total points possible and multiplying the results by 100.

SCORE: _____

SKILL COMPETENCY ASSESSMENT

| 28-5 Placement of Cement Bases *(corresponds to textbook Procedure 28-15)*

Student's Name _____ Date _____

Instructor's Name _____

SKILL   Routine steps should be followed for all treatment areas to maintain absolute clinical asepsis. The dental assistant is responsible for preparation of equipment and supplies needed for the appointment. Cement bases are mixed to thick putty consistency and placed into the cavity preparation to protect the pulp and provide mechanical support for the restoration. These cement bases are placed on the floor of the cavity preparation to raise the level of the floor of the preparation to the ideal height. The preparation, sensitivity of the pulp, and type of restoration will indicate which cement to use.

PERFORMANCE OBJECTIVE   The student will follow a routine procedure that meets the regulations and the protocol set forth by the dentist and regulatory agencies, keeping in mind that assistants' duties vary from state to state. The assistant may be evaluated by performance, statement, and/or combined responses and action. This procedure is performed by the dentist or an expanded-functions dental assistant. The preparation of the cavity has been completed, and this procedure is part of preparing the tooth for the restoration.

	Self Evaluation	Student Evaluation	Possible Points	Instructor Evaluation	Comments
Equipment and Supplies					
1. Cement base materials, usually powder/liquid			3		
2. Mixing pad			3		
3. Cement spatula			3		
4. Gauze sponges			3		
5. Plastic filling instrument					
6. Explorer or spoon excavator					
Competency Steps					
1. Determine previous treatment and decide where to place base and size of area. Evaluate access and visibility.			3		
2. Prepare preparation area. Remove any debris with air-water syringe and HVE.			3		
3. Prepare cement base materials according to manufacturer's instructions. Mix cement base to thick putty consistency and gather into a small ball.			3		
4. Collect base on the blade of plastic filling instrument. Place base into cavity preparation.			3		
5. Using small condensing end of plastic filling instrument, condense base into place on floor of cavity prep. Continue until sufficient base layer is placed.			3		
6. Evaluate placement. Base should cover floor of cavity preparation, enough room left for restorative materials, should not be on pins or retentive grooves.			3		
7. Remove any excess materials with spoon excavator or explorer.			3		

28-5 continued *(corresponds to textbook Procedure 28-15)*

	Self Evaluation	Student Evaluation	Possible Points	Instructor Evaluation	Comments
8. Clean up mixing materials, remove cement from spatula as soon as possible, and remove paper from pad.			3		

TOTAL POINTS POSSIBLE	36
TOTAL POINTS POSSIBLE—2nd Attempt	34
TOTAL POINTS EARNED	_____

Points assigned reflect importance of step to meeting objective: Important = 1; Essential = 2; Critical = 3. Students will lose 2 points for repeated attempts. Failure results if any of the critical steps are omitted or performed incorrectly. If using a 100-point scale, determine score by dividing points earned by total points possible and multiplying the results by 100.

SCORE: _____

SKILL COMPETENCY ASSESSMENT

28-6 Removal of the Simple Suture and Continuous Simple Sutures
(corresponds to textbook Procedure 28-16)

Student's Name _____ Date _____

Instructor's Name _____

SKILL   Routine steps should be followed for all treatment areas to maintain absolute clinical asepsis. The dental assistant is responsible for preparation of equipment and supplies needed for the appointment. Each type of suture is a specific pattern. To remove the sutures, identify the pattern and determine where the cuts are to be made, then follow the basic criteria to remove the suture from the suture site.

PERFORMANCE OBJECTIVE   The student will follow a routine procedure that meets the regulations and the protocol set forth by the dentist and regulatory agencies, keeping in mind that assistants' duties vary from state to state. The assistant may be evaluated by performance, statement, and/or combined responses and action. This procedure is performed by the dentist or an expanded-functions dental assistant. The patient returns to the office for suture removal. The dental assistant prepares the materials needed and the patient before beginning the procedure.

	Self Evaluation	Student Evaluation	Possible Points	Instructor Evaluation	Comments
Equipment and Supplies					
1. Basic setup: mouth mirror, explorer, cotton pliers			3		
2. Suture scissors			3		
3. Hemostat			3		
4. Gauze sponges			3		
5. Air-water syringe tip, HVE tip			3		
Competency Steps					
1. Using cotton pliers, gently lift suture away from tissues.			3		
2. Take suture scissors and cut thread below knot, close to tissue.			3		
3. Secure knot with cotton pliers and gently pull, lifting suture out of tissues.			3		
4. Place suture on gauze sponge.			3		
5. For continuous simple suture, cut each suture and remove individually (begin with one end and proceed with each suture stitch).			3		
6. Loosen suture with cotton pliers and while still holding suture thread with cotton pliers, cut thread close to tissue.			3		
7. As each suture is removed, place on gauze sponge so it can be counted when finished with procedure.			3		

TOTAL POINTS POSSIBLE   36

TOTAL POINTS POSSIBLE—2nd Attempt   34

TOTAL POINTS EARNED   _____

Points assigned reflect importance of step to meeting objective: Important = 1; Essential = 2; Critical = 3. Students will lose 2 points for repeated attempts. Failure results if any of the critical steps are omitted or performed incorrectly. If using a 100-point scale, determine score by dividing points earned by total points possible and multiplying the results by 100.

SCORE: _____

SKILL COMPETENCY ASSESSMENT

28-8 Placing Enamel Sealants *(corresponds to textbook Procedure 28-20)*

Student's Name _____ Date _____

Instructor's Name _____

SKILL   Routine steps should be followed for all treatment areas to maintain absolute clinical asepsis. The dental assistant is responsible for preparation of equipment and supplies needed for the appointment. The dentist will diagnose which teeth need enamel sealants after a thorough examination, including radiographs. The sealant kits are usually supplied with everything needed when applying the sealants.

PERFORMANCE OBJECTIVE   The student will follow a routine procedure that meets the regulations and the protocol set forth by the dentist and regulatory agencies, keeping in mind that assistants' duties vary from state to state. The assistant may be evaluated by performance, statement, and/or combined responses and action. This procedure is performed by the dental assistant, hygienist, or dentist depending on the state Dental Practice Act. Before the sealant is placed, the tooth or teeth are polished with a rubber cup. Equipment and supplies for the preparation of the tooth/teeth and the actual sealant procedure are listed.

	Self Evaluation	Student Evaluation	Possible Points	Instructor Evaluation	Comments
Equipment and Supplies					
1. Basic setup: mouth mirror, explorer, cotton pliers			3		
2. Air-water syringe tip, HVE tips, and saliva ejector			3		
3. Rubber cup			3		
4. Low-speed handpiece with right angle attachment			3		
5. Flour of pumice or prophy paste without fluoride			3		
6. Dental dam setup or Garmer cotton roll holders and short and long cotton rolls			3		
7. Etchant/conditioner			3		
8. Sealant material:					
A. Base material and catalyst (self-cure)			3		
B. Base material (light cure)			3		
9. Applicators (brush, small cotton pellets, or syringe) for etchant and sealant			3		
10. Sealant dappen dish			3		
11. Light-curing unit			3		
12. Articulating paper and forceps			3		
13. Assorted burs and/or stones			3		
14. Floss			3		
Competency Steps					
1. Polish occlusal surface of teeth to receive sealant:					
A. Use flour of pumice or non-fluoride prophy paste with rubber cup or bristle brush			3		
B. Clean occlusal surfaces			3		
C. Rinse teeth and dry thoroughly			3		

28-8 continued *(corresponds to textbook Procedure 28-20)*

	Self Evaluation	Student Evaluation	Possible Points	Instructor Evaluation	Comments
D. Check pits and fissures with explorer			3		
E. Rinse and dry again			3		
2. Isolation:					
A. Dental dam			3		
B. Cotton rolls and/or Garmer clamps (long or short cotton rolls)			3		
3. Dry and etch:					
A. After tooth/teeth isolated, dry			3		
B. Apply etchant—follow manufacturer's directions (use applicator, apply to occlusal surface, into pits and fissures and two-thirds up cuspid incline, using dabbing motion while applying sealant)			3		
C. Time usually 60 seconds			3		
4. Rinse for twenty to thirty seconds. Use evacuator tip to remove remaining acid and water (reisolate with dry cotton rolls if this method was used).			3		
5. Dry all etched surfaces and examine appearance (twenty to thirty seconds). It should appear dull and chalky white (if not, etch again for fifteen to thirty seconds).			3		
6. Apply sealant material. Applicator tip or an explorer can be used to move sealant, prevent air bubbles and reach desired thickness (follow manufacturer's directions to prepare and apply).			3		
7. Curing the sealant:					
A. Allow self-curing sealants to set (polymerize) by manufacturer's direction			3		
B. For light-cured sealants, hold curing light 2 mm directly above occlusal surface, expose for appropriate time (materials differ—range twenty to sixty seconds), use tinted protective eyewear during curing process			3		
8. Evaluate the sealant:					
A. With explorer, check whether sealant hardened and smooth			3		
B. If irregularities or voids, repeat process to properly seal areas			3		
C. If surface free from saliva, additional sealant can be added without etching tooth first			3		
D. If saliva has contacted tooth, process must be completely repeated			3		
9. Rinse the sealant after it has set. Rinse or wipe surface with moist cotton roll/pellet to remove air-inhibited layer.			3		
10. Finishing the sealant:					
A. Remove cotton rolls or dental dam			3		

28-8 continued *(corresponds to textbook Procedure 28-20)*

	Self Evaluation	Student Evaluation	Possible Points	Instructor Evaluation	Comments
B. Check contact with dental floss			3		
C. Dry teeth and place articulating paper to evaluate any high spots			3		
D. Occlusion reduction—as needed by markings			3		
11. Apply fluoride:					
A. Apply fluoride to sealed tooth/teeth etched but not sealed			3		
B. Sealants recorded on patient's chart			3		
C. Instruct patient about checking sealants every six months			3		

TOTAL POINTS POSSIBLE   126

TOTAL POINTS POSSIBLE—2nd Attempt   124

TOTAL POINTS EARNED   _____

Points assigned reflect importance of step to meeting objective: Important = 1; Essential = 2; Critical = 3. Students will lose 2 points for repeated attempts. Failure results if any of the critical steps are omitted or performed incorrectly. If using a 100-point scale, determine score by dividing points earned by total points possible and multiplying the results by 100.

SCORE: _____

SKILL COMPETENCY ASSESSMENT

28-9 In-Office Bleaching for Vital Teeth *(corresponds to textbook Procedure 28-22)*

Student's Name _____ Date _____

Instructor's Name _____

SKILL   Routine steps should be followed for all treatment areas to maintain absolute clinical asepsis. The dental assistant is responsible for preparation of equipment and supplies needed for the appointment. Bleaching vital teeth in the office involves the application of bleaching liquids or gels, often with the application of heat and a curing light.

PERFORMANCE OBJECTIVE   The student will follow a routine procedure that meets the regulations and the protocol set forth by the dentist and regulatory agencies, keeping in mind that assistants' duties vary from state to state. The assistant may be evaluated by performance, statement, and/or combined responses and action. This procedure is performed by the dentist in the dental office. The procedure is explained to the patient with the possible outcomes.

	Self Evaluation	Student Evaluation	Possible Points	Instructor Evaluation	Comments
Equipment and Supplies					
1. Protective gel			3		
2. Waxed dental floss			3		
3. High-speed handpiece and assorted burs			3		
4. Low-speed handpiece			3		
5. Prophy brush			3		
6. Cement base materials			3		
7. Bleaching materials			3		
8. Heat source			3		
9. Temporary coverage and cement			3		
10. Finishing burs			3		
Competency Steps					
1. Procedure is explained and videos, photos, and pamphlets may be available for patient. Teeth and surrounding tissues examined.			3		
2. Isolation:					
A. Cover all surrounding tissues with protective gel			3		
B. Placement of dental dam and ligature waxed dental floss on designated tooth/teeth (pull floss toward the cervix and secure)					
C. Adding additional gel to seal dam			3		
3. Polish crowns of teeth to remove plaque debris that might interfere with bleaching process (prophy paste or flour of pumice).			3		
4. Bleaching procedure:					
A. Material mixed to thick consistency (follow manufacturer's instructions for specific steps to use)			3		
B. Place on facial and lingual surfaces of tooth or in a tray			3		

28-9 continued *(corresponds to textbook Procedure 28-22)*

	Self Evaluation	Student Evaluation	Possible Points	Instructor Evaluation	Comments
C. Bleaching heat and/or light source (approximately thirty minutes)			3		
D. No-heat materials are applied every ten minutes, with fresh materials mixed each time for three to four applications			3		
E. Rinse and evacuate between each application			3		
F. To remove bulk of bleaching gel			3		
5. Remove isolation materials:					
A. Thoroughly rinse area			3		
B. Cut ligatures and interseptal dam			3		
C. Remove dental dam from patient's mouth			3		
D. Rinse again			3		
E. Remove any protective gel with floss and wet gauze			3		
6. Polish teeth with composite resin polishing cup or fluoride prophy paste.			3		
7. Examine area, check patient's tissues. Patient is instructed to avoid substances that may stain teeth and is warned that teeth may be sensitive following bleaching (usually three appointments, one to two weeks apart arc required to reach desired shade).			3		

TOTAL POINTS POSSIBLE   84

TOTAL POINTS POSSIBLE—2nd Attempt   82

TOTAL POINTS EARNED   _____

Points assigned reflect importance of step to meeting objective: Important = 1; Essential = 2; Critical = 3. Students will lose 2 points for repeated attempts. Failure results if any of the critical steps are omitted or performed incorrectly. If using a 100-point scale, determine score by dividing points earned by total points possible and multiplying the results by 100.

SCORE: _____

Dental Office Management

OBJECTIVES

The student should strive to meet the following objectives and demonstrate an understanding of the facts and principles presented in this chapter:

1. Identify the dental office staff and their areas of responsibility.
2. Identify marketing ideas for dentistry.
3. Outline the proper procedure for answering an incoming call.
4. Describe the information every message should contain.
5. Describe telephone and business office technology and its uses.
6. Give examples of the ways in which computers are used in the dental office.
7. Explain how database management concepts can be used in the dental office.
8. Explain why ergonomics is important at a computer workstation.
9. Explain ways in which effective patient scheduling can be accomplished in the dental office.
10. Identify the equipment needed for record management.
11. Define key terms related to accounts receivable.
12. Identify computerized and manual systems for management of patient accounts.
13. Identify accounts payable expenses that the dental practice is responsible for.

SUMMARY

The dental reception area needs to be an environment in which all patients feel welcome and comfortable. Today, dentistry can be a positive experience, and the dental treatment can be pain free. That image is developed when the patient first steps into the reception area. The patients may not realize consciously the message that is being received, but the dental office should present an atmosphere that relieves feelings of anxiety.

The front office staff has changed dramatically in recent years. All of the individuals in the front office need knowledge of business machines such as computers, fax machines, and copy machines. These individuals must be organized, have a knowledge of dental treatments, and have good communication and problem-solving skills.

Marketing is also an important part of the dental profession. A dental office is a business as well as a health-care facility. Dental assistants, along with all the members of the dental team, need to be involved in marketing the practice and the dentistry that can be provided.

KEY TERMS

accounts payable
accounts receivable
Americans with Disabilities Act
check register
computerized systems
down time
ergonomics
etiquette

expendable
facsimile
file folder
gross income
hardware
net income
non-expendable
overlap of time

overtime
packing slip
personal computers (PCs)
petty cash
software
tickler file
usual, reasonable, and
    customary fee

EXERCISES AND ACTIVITIES

1. This act, which was passed by Congress, mandates that individuals with disabilities are to have accessibility to health-care facilities having more than fifteen employees. _____
   A. External marketing
   B. Ergonomics consultant
   C. Onsight technology education services
   D. Americans with Disabilities

2. Which accounting term indicates the money owed to the practice? _____
   A. Accounts payable
   B. Accounts receivable
   C. Inventory
   D. Non-expendable

3. Which accounting term indicates the amount the practice owes others? _____
   A. Gross income
   B. Accounts payable
   C. Accounts receivable
   D. Petty cash

4. Which one of the following is not a part of a computer function? _____
   A. Spreadsheet
   B. Word processing
   C. Cellular phones
   D. Database management

5. The computer program or set of instructions that tells the hardware what to do is called _____
   A. hardware.   C. facsimile.
   B. software.   D. tickler file.

6. The goal of the receptionist is to fill the appointment book with patient care. Time in the appointment book that is not scheduled is called _____
   A. down time.
   B. overtime.
   C. overlap time.
   D. tickler file.

7. In scheduling, when patient treatment time goes beyond the estimated time frame, it is called _____
   A. down time.
   B. overtime.
   C. overlap time.
   D. tickler file.

8. _____ time occurs when the dentist or auxiliary is required to be in two places at the same time.
   A. Down   C. Overlap of
   B. Over   D. Tickler

9. A well-organized office will have what file to serve as a reminder of any action that needs to be taken in the future? _____
   A. Recall   C. Facsimile
   B. Tickler   D. Archival

10. A fee schedule is used to define what patients will be charged for each service. It is referred to as _____
    A. professional courtesy.
    B. usual, responsible, and customary fee.
    C. insurance.
    D. record management.

11. When you subtract the accounts payable from the gross income, you identify the _____
    A. overhead.
    B. net income.
    C. gross income.
    D. petty cash.

12. There are several inventory records systems that can be used to keep track of supplies. Supplies that are retained in the office for long periods of time are referred to as _____
    A. non-expendable.
    B. expendable.
    C. shelf life.
    D. variable.

13. When supplies are shipped, the supplier will enclose a list of items included. When receiving supplies, you will check this list and note any discrepancies. This list is called a _____
    A. statement.
    B. credit slip.
    C. back order slip.
    D. packing slip.

14. As part of accounts payable, this record reflects all deposits and checks made from the account and is called the _____
    A. bank statement.
    B. check register.
    C. payroll.
    D. credit slip.

15. Which of the following are basic telephone techniques? _____
    1. Enunciate, speak clearly, and articulate carefully
    2. State who the message is for
    3. Speak at a normal rate of speed
    4. Ask what action is required
    5. Always use telephone etiquette, good manners
    6. Record date and time call received

    A. 1, 2, 6
    B. 1, 3, 6
    C. 1, 3, 5
    D. 1, 4, 6

16. As part of the business office equipment, answering systems may include which of the following? _____
    1. Voice mail
    2. E-mail
    3. Word processing
    4. Fax
    5. Graphics
    6. Database management

    A. 3, 4, 6
    B. 1, 2, 6
    C. 2, 3, 4
    D. 1, 2, 4

17. The total accounts receivable is calculated as the _____
    A. gross income.
    B. net income.

SKILL COMPETENCY ASSESSMENT

29-1 Balancing the Day Sheets and the End-of-the-Month Figures
(corresponds to textbook Procedure 29-4)

Student's Name _____ Date _____

Instructor's Name _____

SKILL The accounts receivable of the dental office encompasses the money owed to the practice. The bookkeeping in this area must be accurate and carries with it a great responsibility. This position may be occupied by the receptionist or the business assistant. All transactions, payments, adjustments, and charges must be handled in a safe and professional manner.

PERFORMANCE OBJECTIVE The student will follow a routine procedure that meets the protocol set forth by the dentist and office staff. The assistant may be evaluated by performance, statement, and/or combined responses and action. The dental receptionist or office business assistant balances the day sheets daily and totals the day sheets at the end of the month or prior to patient statements being sent out.

	Self Evaluation	Student Evaluation	Possible Points	Instructor Evaluation	Comments
Equipment and Supplies					
1. Pegboard			3		
2. Day sheets totaled for month			3		
3. Ledger cards for all patients in storage file			3		
4. Calculator with tape that records entries			3		
Competency Steps					
1. First step in balancing day sheets, total each column and place total in spaces provided at bottom of page in "Totals this page" (this section is identified as section 4).			3		
2. Column totals are added to "Previous page" totals and number is placed in "Month to Date" total spaces.			3		
3. Totals are verified in "Proof of Posting" box in section 5 (where total of column D is added to column A and subtotaled).			3		
4. Once proof of posting is complete, accounts receivable control can be totaled:			3		
A. Add total of column A to previous day's total			3		
B. Subtract columns B1 and B2 from subtotal			3		
C. True balance of accounts receivable			3		
5. Next total up amounts owed on ledger cards (use tape for verification).			3		
6. If total of ledger cards balances with total on day sheet, accounts receivable is balanced (not balanced, recheck figures and find missing amount).			3		

29-1 continued *(corresponds to textbook Procedure 29-4)*

	Self Evaluation	Student Evaluation	Possible Points	Instructor Evaluation	Comments
7. Statements can be sent out after account receivable is balanced.			3		

TOTAL POINTS POSSIBLE		42
TOTAL POINTS POSSIBLE—2nd Attempt		40
TOTAL POINTS EARNED		_____

Points assigned reflect importance of step to meeting objective: Important = 1; Essential = 2; Critical = 3. Students will lose 2 points for repeated attempts. Failure results if any of the critical steps are omitted or performed incorrectly. If using a 100-point scale, determine score by dividing points earned by total points possible and multiplying the results by 100.

SCORE: _____

SKILL COMPETENCY ASSESSMENT

29-2 Preparing a Deposit Slip *(corresponds to textbook Procedure 29-5)*

Student's Name _____ Date _____

Instructor's Name _____

SKILL   The dental receptionist or the office business assistant is responsible for recording payments promptly onto the ledgers and into the bookkeeping system. Totals are deposited into the bank daily.

PERFORMANCE OBJECTIVE   The student will follow a routine procedure that meets the protocol set forth by the dentist and office staff. The assistant may be evaluated by performance, statement, and/or combined responses and action. The dental receptionist or office business assistant creates the deposit slip and either takes it to the bank or the dentist takes it to the bank to be deposited. Deposits are normally made in person or placed in the night deposit.

	Self Evaluation	Student Evaluation	Possible Points	Instructor Evaluation	Comments
Equipment and Supplies					
1. Deposit slip			3		
2. Cash and checks received for that day			3		
3. Office stamp for endorsing checks			3		
4. Envelop in which to place the deposit slip, checks, and cash			3		
Competency Steps					
1. Place date on deposit slip.			3		
2. Separate currency (coin, paper money) from checks.			3		
3. Tally coins, place total sum in designated space on deposit slip.			3		
4. Tally paper money and place total sum in designated space on deposit slip.			3		
5. On back of deposit slip, list each check separately, listing patient's last name and amount of check in space provided in right-hand column.			3		
6. Total list amounts from checks on the back of deposit slip and place this sum in area on the front of check slip in space identified as checks.			3		
7. Total currency (both coins, paper money) and check amount and place this sum at bottom of deposit slip under total (amount should total the total identified on payments column on day sheet; one other way to further check the total is accurate is to add up coins, paper money, and each check—this verifies sum is correct).			3		

29-2 continued *(corresponds to textbook Procedure 29-5)*

	Self Evaluation	Student Evaluation	Possible Points	Instructor Evaluation	Comments
8. Enter date and the amount of the deposit into checkbook stub.			3		

TOTAL POINTS POSSIBLE   36

TOTAL POINTS POSSIBLE—2nd Attempt   34

TOTAL POINTS EARNED   _____

Points assigned reflect importance of step to meeting objective: Important = 1; Essential = 2; Critical = 3. Students will lose 2 points for repeated attempts. Failure results if any of the critical steps are omitted or performed incorrectly. If using a 100-point scale, determine score by dividing points earned by total points possible and multiplying the results by 100.

SCORE: _____

SKILL COMPETENCY ASSESSMENT

29-3 Reordering Supplies *(corresponds to textbook Procedure 29-6)*

Student's Name _____ Date _____

Instructor's Name _____

SKILL The reordering point ensures that an adequate supply is available taking into consideration the lead time and the rate of use for the product. There are several inventory records systems that can be utilized in the dental office to keep track of the supplies. The goal of any system is that the supplies are available when they are needed.

PERFORMANCE OBJECTIVE The student will follow a routine procedure that meets the protocol set forth by the dentist and office staff. The assistant may be evaluated by performance, statement, and/or combined responses and action. The dental assistant may be assigned specifically to order supplies, or this task may be shared by several auxiliaries.

	Self Evaluation	Student Evaluation	Possible Points	Instructor Evaluation	Comments
Equipment and Supplies					
Red Flag Reorder Tag System					
1. Red flag reorder tags that have surfaced for reordering			3		
2. Telephone			3		
3. Index card with order information			3		
Electronic Bar Code System					
1. Bar code wand			3		
2. Telephone			3		
Competency Steps					
Red Flag Reorder Tag System					
1. Gather red flags that indicate items that require reordering.			3		
2. Check index card to obtain ordering information for each item.			3		
3. Place an indicator in upper-right corner to indicate this item is to be ordered immediately.			3		
4. After item is ordered, place indicator in upper-left corner until product arrives.			3		
5. When item arrives, remove indicator from tag.			3		
6. Place most recently received items to back of supply (using older materials first).			3		
7. Place red flag ordering tag on minimum quantity needed in stock before reordering must be accomplished again.			3		
Electronic Bar Code System					
1. Identify items that require reordering (this system is used for commonly ordered items).			3		

29-3 continued *(corresponds to textbook Procedure 29-6)*

	Self Evaluation	Student Evaluation	Possible Points	Instructor Evaluation	Comments
2. Obtain book that has product information and bar codes identified.			3		
3. Use bar code wand to input items needed, run wand over bar codes of items needing ordering.			3		
4. Indicate on transmitter the number of items needed (order is then transmitted directly to dental supply company for ordering).			3		
5. Place date on listed items and indicate the number that have been ordered.					

TOTAL POINTS POSSIBLE   51

TOTAL POINTS POSSIBLE—2nd Attempt   49

TOTAL POINTS EARNED   _____

Points assigned reflect importance of step to meeting objective: Important = 1; Essential = 2; Critical = 3. Students will lose 2 points for repeated attempts. Failure results if any of the critical steps are omitted or performed incorrectly. If using a 100-point scale, determine score by dividing points earned by total points possible and multiplying the results by 100.

SCORE: _____

SKILL COMPETENCY ASSESSMENT

29-4 Reconciling a Bank Statement *(corresponds to textbook Procedure 29-7)*

Student's Name _____ Date _____

Instructor's Name _____

SKILL Each month the bank sends a statement showing any transactions that took place within the account during the month. It lists all checks that have cleared the bank, any deposits received by the bank, and any service charges that were deducted from the account. It should be reconciled against the entries made in the dental office check register.

PERFORMANCE OBJECTIVE The student will follow a routine procedure that meets the protocol set forth by the dentist and office staff. The assistant may be evaluated by performance, statement, and/or combined responses and action. The dental receptionist or business assistant will reconcile the bank statement each month.

	Self Evaluation	Student Evaluation	Possible Points	Instructor Evaluation	Comments
Equipment and Supplies					
1. Bank statement			3		
2. Checkbook			3		
3. Calculator			3		
Competency Steps					
1. Make sure all checks and deposits have been added or subtracted from checkbook.			3		
2. Subtract any bank service charge from the last balance listed in checkbook.			3		
3. Check off each listed check in bank statement against checkbook and verify amount listed.			3		
4. Check off each deposit listed in bank statement against checkbook and verify amount listed.			3		
5. On back of bank statement, place ending balance from front of statement in ending balance space on worksheet.			3		
6. List all checks from checkbook that have not cleared bank in section provided on back of worksheet.			3		
7. List all deposits from checkbook that have not been received by bank on space provided on worksheet on back of statement.			3		
8. Total checks not cleared and deposits not received.			3		
9. Subtract checks not received from ending balance on bank statement.			3		
10. Add deposits not received to ending balance on bank statement.			3		
11. Balance should agree with checkbook balance (if any bank charges on statement, make					

29-4 continued *(corresponds to textbook Procedure 9-7)*

	Self Evaluation	Student Evaluation	Possible Points	Instructor Evaluation	Comments
corresponding adjustments in checkbook balance).			3		

TOTAL POINTS POSSIBLE   42

TOTAL POINTS POSSIBLE—2nd Attempt   40

TOTAL POINTS EARNED   _____

Points assigned reflect importance of step to meeting objective: Important = 1; Essential = 2; Critical = 3. Students will lose 2 points for repeated attempts. Failure results if any of the critical steps are omitted or performed incorrectly. If using a 100-point scale, determine score by dividing points earned by total points possible and multiplying the results by 100.

SCORE: _____

Employment Strategies

OBJECTIVES

The student should strive to meet the following objectives and demonstrate an understanding of the facts and principles presented in this chapter:

1. Identify four pathways to obtain DANB certification.
2. Explain how to obtain employment and identify different types of practices.
3. Set goals and identify sources to obtain employment in the dental field.
4. Identify the steps of preparing a cover letter and a résumé.
5. Define how to prepare for the interview.
6. Explain the interview process and identify skills and preparation techniques that will aid in obtaining the job.
7. Identify the skills that a successful dental assistant possesses. Explain how to terminate employment.

SUMMARY

It is important to find employment that will best suit individual needs and that allows for the best possible situation for the dental assistant, employer, and the patients. Before taking the first position available, plan ahead. It may be essential to obtain dental assisting national certification for the state in which employment is sought. National certification for dental assistants is not mandatory in every state, but it assures the patients and the dentist that the assistant has the basic knowledge and background to perform as a professional on the dental team. Make sure that expectations of the job are identified and then try to meet and exceed those if planning to advance. Each dental assistant is responsible for maintaining a positive attitude at work. Set goals to learn new skills and stay abreast of changes in technology and materials. A dental assisting career is very rewarding, both professionally and personally. Be the best dental assistant possible.

KEY TERMS

American Dental Assistants
    Association (ADAA)
American Dental Association (ADA)
Dental Assisting National Board,
    Inc. (DANB)
dental associate
partnership

EXERCISES AND ACTIVITIES

1. A dentist may hire another dentist under a contractual agreement; this hired dentist is a dental _____.
   A. partner.
   B. solo.
   C. associate.
   D. group.

2. Any number of dentists (both general and specialty) can share a building and still remain independent. This type of dental office is called a _____
   A. specialty practice.
   B. partnership.
   C. group practice.
   D. solo practice.

3. In which employment choice does the dental assistant treat patients who are eligible to receive dental care at a reduced rate? _____
   A. Group practice
   B. Government clinics
   C. Solo practice
   D. Insurance programmer

4. In which employment choice must the assistant obtain employment through the Civil Service office in order to assist the dentists on staff? _____
   A. Federal
   B. State
   C. Dental school
   D. Veterans' hospital

5. The dental assistant will need to research which of the following areas to locate employment and open positions? _____
   A. Dental supply houses
   B. Classified section of daily paper
   C. Local dental society
   D. All of the above

6. One of the goals of the job search is to seek and obtain successful employment. Which of the following would indicate an office that would be enjoyable to work in? _____
   A. Goods and supplies on hand
   B. Good advertisement in paper
   C. Practice seems most interesting
   D. Employees would not talk to me

7. A portfolio can be prepared for the interview and would include which of the following? _____
   A. Letters of recommendation
   B. Copies of certification
   C. Radiographs taken
   D. All of the above

8. Qualities that a dentist looks for in a dental assistant include which of the following? _____
   A. Good clinical skills
   B. Team player
   C. Good interpersonal skills
   D. Willing to learn
   E. All of the above

9. To terminate employment in your office, provide the employer _____ notice.
   A. no
   B. two weeks'
   C. one week's
   D. two days'

10. Eligibility for national certification can be obtained by which of the following criteria for Pathway I? _____
    1. High school graduation or equivalent
    2. Current CPR card, health-care provider level
    3. Verification of dentist employer
    4. Graduate of an accredited dental assistant or dental hygiene program
    5. Application fee
    6. 3,500 hours of employment

    A. 1, 2, 5
    B. 2, 3, 5
    C. 2, 4, 5
    D. 1, 5, 6

11. In development of a cover letter, there is a standard format that follows a specific order. Place the following items in the order in which they would appear in a cover letter. _____
    1. Closing ("Sincerely")
    2. Date
    3. Return address
    4. Second paragraph
    5. First paragraph
    6. Inside address
    7. Third paragraph
    8. Salutation ("To whom it may concern")
    9. Enclosure

    A. 3, 2, 6, 8, 5, 4, 7, 1, 9
    B. 8, 2, 3, 5, 4, 7, 1, 6, 9
    C. 2, 3, 8, 5, 4, 7, 1, 6, 9
    D. 6, 2, 3, 8, 4, 5, 7, 1, 9

12. The résumé should fit on one page and follow the standard format. Place the following items in the order in which they would appear in a résumé. _____

    1. Education
    2. Employment history
    3. Career objective
    4. Personal data
    5. References

    A. 3, 4, 2, 1, 5
    B. 4, 1, 3, 2, 5
    C. 3, 4, 1, 2, 5
    D. 4, 3, 1, 2, 5

13. When preparing for the interview, there are several things to think about. Which of the following items will make for a successful interview? _____

    1. Arrive five minutes early
    2. Wear jeans
    3. Smile
    4. Demonstrate good hygiene
    5. Control the interview
    6. Being a good speller is not critical

    A. 1, 3, 5
    B. 1, 3, 4
    C. 2, 5, 6
    D. 1, 2, 4

14. A dental _____ is developed through a legal agreement and makes both dentists responsible for any accounts payable.

    A. associate
    B. partnership

Ethics and Jurisprudence

OBJECTIVES

The student should strive to meet the following objectives and demonstrate an understanding of the facts and principles presented in this chapter:

1. Identify the difference between civil and criminal law.
2. Define the Dental Practice Act and what it covers.
3. Identify who oversees the Dental Practice Act and how licenses for the dental field are obtained.
4. Define expanded functions.
5. Identify the components of a contract.
6. Identify due care and give examples of malpractice and torts.
7. Identify fraud and the service that can be given under the Good Samaritan Law.
8. Identify the four areas of the Americans with Disabilities Act.
9. Identify the responsibilities of the dental team in regard to dental records, implied and informed consent, subpoenas, and the statute of limitations.
10. Define ethics and give examples of the American Dental Association and American Dental Assistants Association principles of ethics.
11. State how dentistry follows ethical principles in regard to advertising, professional fees and charges, and professional responsibilities and rights.

SUMMARY

Each dental team member is faced with daily decisions that require judgments regarding legal and ethical principles. Maintaining professional ethical standards at all times is essential. The consequences for not doing what should be legally done or doing what should not be done can include fines or imprisonment. A license is granted to protect the public from unqualified individuals providing dental treatment. Some states require dental assistants to become licensed to perform specific dental tasks. The expanded functions are most often specified in the Dental Practice Act according to how they are to be delegated. They may be stipulated for general supervision, which means that the procedure authorized in the Dental Practice Act can be legally performed on a patient of record by the dental assistant under the general supervision of the dentist, or they may be specified to be delegated under direct supervision. The dental assistant must thoroughly understand the law in order to protect the patient, the dentist, and the profession. Dental health care continues to change and the assistant must understand how the law affects these changes.

KEY TERMS

abandonment	civil law	dental jurisprudence	expanded functions	informed consent
Americans with	contract	Dental Practice Act	expressed contract	malpractice
Disabilities Act	contract law	Doctrine of	Good Samaritan	reciprocity
assault	criminal law	Respondeat	Law	statutes
battery	defamation of	Superior	implied consent	tort
breach of contract	character	ethics	implied contract	

EXERCISES AND ACTIVITIES

1. The area of law that governs dentistry is _____
   A. civil law.
   B. criminal law.
   C. dental jurisprudence.
   D. common law.

2. The area of law that clearly defines moral judgment is _____
   A. civil law.
   B. criminal law.
   C. common law.
   D. ethics.

3. In each state, what is (are) enacted by each legislative body to make rules and regulations? _____
   A. State Board of Dentistry
   B. Statutes
   C. Dental Practice Act
   D. Reciprocity

4. What gives states guidelines for eligibility for licensing and identifies the grounds by which this license can be suspended or repealed? _____
   A. Dental jurisprudence
   B. Dental Practice Act
   C. State Board of Dentistry
   D. Statutes

5. Delegated functions that require increased responsibility and skill are called _____
   A. expanded functions.
   B. dental jurisprudence.
   C. laws.
   D. contracts.

6. In some states, an individual who has passed the requirements for one state may apply for a _____ agreement in another state and be allowed to perform dental skills without taking a written or clinical exam again.
   A. contract   C. reciprocity
   B. consent   D. malpractice

7. Expanded functions are specific advanced functions that require increased skill and responsibility. Like all functions the auxiliary performs, the expanded functions fall under the _____, which translated means "Let the master answer."
   A. American Dental Association
   B. Dental Practice Act
   C. Good Samaritan Law
   D. Doctrine of Respondeat Superior

8. A binding agreement between two or more people is called _____
   A. a contract.
   B. informed consent.
   C. implied consent.
   D. a tort.

9. A contract that can be written or verbal and that describes specifically what each party in the contract will do is called _____
   A. informed consent.
   B. an expressed contract.
   C. a breach of contract.
   D. a termination contract.

10. If a contract is broken, this is called _____
    A. a breach of contract.
    B. an expressed contract.
    C. a patient discharge.
    D. noncompliant.

11. What is the legal term used when dentists fail to notify a patient that they can no longer provide services? _____
    A. Noncompliant   C. Negligence
    B. Due care   D. Abandonment

12. The dentist and the dental team members have the responsibility and duty to perform due care in treating all patients. Failure to do this is called _____
    A. assault.   C. malpractice.
    B. sufficient care. D. abandonment.

13. A tort law protects an individual from causing injury to another person's reputation, name, or character. This injury is called _____
    A. invasion of privacy.
    B. defamation of character.
    C. assault and battery.
    D. fraud.

14. The area of law covering any wrongful act that is a breach in due care and where injury has resulted from the action is called _____
    A. malpractice   C. civil law
    B. ethics   D. torts

15. If a child was refusing treatment and the dental personnel threatened and restrained the child without parental consent, what charges could be brought? _____
    A. Civil law
    B. Criminal law
    C. Assault and battery
    D. Invasion of privacy

16. When care is given without intent to do bodily harm and without being compensated for this care, this is called _____
    A. Americans with Disabilities Act.
    B. invasion of privacy.
    C. Doctrine of Respondeat Superior.
    D. a Good Samaritan act.

17. What national mandate stipulates that individuals not be discriminated against because of their disabilities? _____
    A. American Dental Association Principles of Ethics
    B. Statute of limitations
    C. Americans with Disabilities Act
    D. Doctrine of Respondeat Superior

18. Each patient has the right to know and understand any procedure that is performed. The form that patients sign, indicating they understand and accept treatment, is called _____
    A. an expressed contract.
    B. an implied contract.
    C. informed consent.
    D. implied consent.

19. When a dentist sits down and the patient opens his or her mouth, what type of consent does this indicate? _____
    A. Informed consent
    B. Implied contract
    C. Implied consent
    D. Expressed contract

20. In the dental care setting, what is the most frequently exercised law? _____
    A. Civil law
    B. Criminal law
    C. Common law
    D. Ethics

21. Which of the following areas are referred to in the Americans with Disabilities Act?_____
    1. Immunity while providing emergency treatment
    2. Disabled are provided access to public services
    3. Telecommunication services to the hearing and speech impaired
    4. Unwanted hug without consent
    5. Threat of unprivileged touching
    6. Employment discrimination due to disability

    A. 1, 4, 5
    B. 2, 4, 5
    C. 2, 3, 6
    D. 1, 2, 6

22. Examples of the American Dental Association Principles of Ethics include which of the following?_____
    1. Advertising
    2. Professional fees
    3. Service to the public and quality of care
    4. Education
    5. Research and development
    6. Enhancing personal gain

    A. 1, 2, 6
    B. 2, 4, 5
    C. 3, 4, 5
    D. 3, 4, 6

CHAPTER 1
Introduction to the Dental Profession
1. E 2. C 3. B 4. C 5. B
6. C 7. C 8. B 9. C 10. C
11. D 12. B 13. E 14. A

CHAPTER 2
Oral Health and Nutrition
1. D 2. D 3. C 4. C 5. C
6. D 7. E 8. C 9. B 10. D
11. D 12. D 13. B 14. E 15. A
16. B 17. A 18. D 19. A 20. C
21. D 22. C 23. A 24. B 25. E
26. D

CHAPTER 3
General Anatomy and Physiology
1. B 2. B 3. B 4. D 5. C
6. B 7. D 8. D 9. B 10. E
11. A 12. E 13. D 14. E 15. B
16. B 17. D 18. D 19. A 20. B
21. C 22. B 23. D 24. C 25. A
26. D 27. B 28. A 29. D 30. B
31. D 32. A 33. B 34. A 35. B
36. C 37. D 38. A 39. B 40. A
41. D 42. D 43. D 44. D

CHAPTER 4
Head and Neck Anatomy
1. A 2. D 3. D 4. C 5. E
6. B 7. D 8. A 9. B 10. A
11. D 12. A 13. D 14. B 15. B
16. A 17. B 18. B 19. B 20. C
21. A 22. C 23. B 24. B 25. B
26. C 27. D 28. D 29. A 30. B
31. A 32. B 33. D 34. D 35. B
36. A 37. D 38. A 39. B 40. D
41. D 42. D 43. A 44. E 45. D
46. B 47. C 48. A 49. D 50. D
51. A 52. B

CHAPTER 5
Embryology and Histology
1. D 2. D 3. B 4. B 5. C
6. A 7. E 8. B 9. B 10. C
11. D 12. C 13. A 14. B 15. C
16. B 17. E 18. B 19. C 20. C
21. D 22. E 23. A 24. B 25. D
26. A 27. D 28. D 29. C 30. E
31. D 32. B 33. A 34. B 35. D
36. B 37. C 38. C 39. C 40. A
41. B 42. C 43. A 44. D 45. B
46. B 47. D 48. E 49. B 50. D
51. D 52. A 53. C 54. A 55. B
56. C 57. A 58. D 59. B

CHAPTER 6
Tooth Morphology
1. C 2. B 3. C 4. B 5. B
6. B 7. D 8. A 9. C 10. B
11. D 12. B 13. E 14. A 15. C
16. D

CHAPTER 7
Dental Charting
1. D 2. B 3. A 4. E 5. D
6. B 7. C 8. D 9. B 10. D
11. A 12. B 13. B 14. C 15. D
16. D 17. C 18. C 19. C 20. B
21. A 22. D 23. D 24. A 25. B
26. E 27. C 28. C 29. A 30. B
31. E 32. D 33. B 34. A 35. C

CHAPTER 8
Microbiology
1. B 2. A 3. B 4. C 5. D
6. B 7. B 8. A 9. C 10. B
11. D 12. A 13. B 14. C 15. A
16. B 17. D 18. E 19. C 20. C
21. B 22. C 23. D 24. B 25. D
26. C 27. D 28. C 29. B 30. B
31. B 32. C 33. B 34. B 35. A
36. D 37. B 38. B 39. C 40. C
41. C 42. D 43. B 44. B 45. B
46. C 47. A 48. E 49. A 50. D
51. C 52. B 53. C 54. E 55. A
56. B 57. D

CHAPTER 9
Infection Control
1. D 2. A 3. D 4. C 5. A
6. B 7. A 8. B 9. D 10. B
11. A 12. C 13. C 14. A 15. E
16. B 17. B 18. D 19. A 20. D
21. B 22. C 23. E 24. A 25. C
26. D 27. A 28. B 29. D 30. C
31. C 32. C 33. D 34. C 35. B
36. B 37. B 38. A 39. A 40. C
41. D 42. A 43. E 44. B 45. D
46. A 47. B 48. C 49. C 50. D
51. A 52. E 53. B

CHAPTER 10
Management of Hazardous Materials
1. D 2. B 3. A 4. D 5. B
6. D 7. C 8. E 9. C 10. A
11. B 12. D 13. B 14. D 15. C
16. C 17. B 18. D 19. C 20. D
21. E 22. A 23. B 24. B 25. D
26. A 27. C

CHAPTER 11
Preparation for Patient Care
1. B 2. D 3. A 4. B 5. B
6. E 7. C 8. D 9. A 10. D
11. C 12. B 13. E 14. C 15. B
16. B 17. D 18. C 19. D 20. B
21. D 22. B 23. B 24. A 25. A
26. B 27. D 28. A 29. C 30. D
31. C 32. B 33. A 34. B 35. C
36. D 37. A 38. B 39. E 40. D
41. A 42. C

CHAPTER 12
Pharmacology
1. C 2. B 3. D 4. C 5. D
6. A 7. D 8. C 9. D 10. C
11. C 12. D 13. C 14. D 15. B
16. A 17. A 18. B 19. C 20. B
21. D 22. A 23. D 24. E 25. A
26. B 27. C 28. B 29. C 30. D
31. A 32. C 33. D 34. B 35. A

CHAPTER 13
Emergency Management
1. D 2. E 3. C 4. B 5. D
6. D 7. A 8. C 9. B 10. A
11. B 12. B 13. D 14. A 15. B
16. C 17. B 18. C 19. C 20. D
21. D 22. B 23. C 24. D 25. C
26. B 27. A 28. C 29. A 30. B
31. B 32. C 33. D 34. C 35. E
36. A 37. B 38. C 39. D 40. E
41. B 42. A 43. D 44. C 45. B
46. A 47. E 48. C 49. A 50. B
51. D

CHAPTER 14
Introduction to Chairside Assisting
1. C 2. D 3. B 4. D 5. B
6. A 7. B 8. C 9. C 10. E
11. A 12. B 13. D 14. A 15. E
16. D 17. C 18. E 19. A 20. B
21. B 22. C 23. A 24. A 25. B
26. A 27. B 28. C 29. D 30. B

CHAPTER 15
Chairside Instruments and Tray Systems

1. A	2. B	3. D	4. C	5. B
6. C	7. D	8. C	9. D	10. C
11. B	12. C	13. B	14. B	15. C
16. C	17. A	18. B	19. C	20. B
21. C	22. C	23. B	24. B	25. C
26. B	27. C	28. C	29. D	30. B
31. A	32. C	33. D	34. A	35. C
36. B	37. B	38. D	39. B	40. D
41. C	42. C	43. C	44. A	45. B
46. C	47. D	48. E	49. A	50. D
51. C	52. B	53. B	54. E	55. A
56. D	57. C	58. B	59. C	60. A
61. C	62. D	63. A	64. E	65. B
66. A				

CHAPTER 16
Management of Pain and Anxiety

1. C	2. D	3. B	4. C	5. B
6. C	7. D	8. B	9. C	10. C
11. B	12. B	13. D	14. D	15. D
16. D	17. C	18. C	19. B	20. B
21. D	22. D	23. D	24. D	25. A
26. B	27. B	28. A	29. B	30. B
31. B	32. D	33. C	34. A	35. B
36. D	37. E	38. B	39. C	40. A

CHAPTER 17
Radiology

1. B	2. C	3. A	4. D	5. A
6. D	7. D	8. B	9. B	10. D
11. C	12. A	13. B	14. A	15. C
16. D	17. B	18. A	19. B	20. A
21. C	22. A	23. B	24. B	25. D
26. A	27. D	28. C	29. B	30. B
31. B	32. B	33. A	34. B	35. C
36. A	37. B	38. B	39. C	40. B
41. D	42. A	43. D	44. A	45. B
46. E	47. C	48. E	49. D	50. B
51. A	52. C	53. C	54. A	55. D
56. B	57. D			

CHAPTER 18
Endodontics

1. D	2. B	3. C	4. B	5. C
6. D	7. A	8. B	9. E	10. B
11. C	12. C	13. B	14. D	15. C
16. D	17. D	18. D	19. C	20. B
21. B	22. A	23. B	24. A	25. B
26. A	27. B	28. A	29. B	30. B
31. A				

CHAPTER 19
Oral and Maxillofacial Surgery

1. D	2. B	3. B	4. C	5. D
6. D	7. B	8. C	9. C	10. D
11. D	12. C	13. C	14. D	15. C
16. D	17. A	18. B	19. B	20. B
21. B	22. B	23. A	24. B	25. B
26. B				

CHAPTER 20
Oral Pathology

1. D	2. D	3. B	4. D	5. D
6. B	7. C	8. A	9. B	10. B
11. D	12. D	13. E	14. C	15. B
16. B	17. B	18. B	19. A	20. C
21. C	22. A	23. C	24. D	25. B
26. B	27. D	28. A	29. C	30. D
31. B	32. C	33. B	34. B	35. A
36. B	37. A	38. B	39. B	40. B
41. A				

CHAPTER 21
Orthodontics

1. D	2. E	3. A	4. C	5. B
6. D	7. E	8. B	9. C	10. B
11. C	12. B	13. D	14. B	15. B
16. C	17. B	18. B	19. B	20. B
21. B	22. A	23. B	24. B	25. A

CHAPTER 22
Pediatric Dentistry

1. B	2. C	3. A	4. D	5. B
6. C	7. B	8. B	9. A	10. C
11. A	12. B	13. B	14. A	15. C
16. D	17. D	18. B		

CHAPTER 23
Periodontics

1. C	2. C	3. B	4. D	5. D
6. A	7. D	8. C	9. C	10. A
11. B	12. B	13. B	14. D	15. C
16. A	17. B	18. C	19. B	20. C
21. A	22. B	23. A	24. B	25. A
26. B	27. B	28. A	29. A	30. B

CHAPTER 24
Fixed Prosthodontics

1. E	2. D	3. A	4. D	5. B
6. B	7. A	8. D	9. C	10. B
11. B	12. B	13. A		

CHAPTER 25
Removable Prosthodontics

1. E	2. A	3. D	4. D	5. B
6. C	7. D	8. C	9. B	10. A
11. C	12. A	13. B	14. A	15. C
16. B				

CHAPTER 26
Chairside Restorative Materials

1. D	2. B	3. A	4. B	5. C
6. A	7. A	8. D	9. C	10. B
11. B	12. A	13. B	14. A	15. B
16. C	17. D	18. A	19. D	20. A
21. B	22. B	23. A	24. C	25. A
26. B	27. C	28. B	29. A	30. A

CHAPTER 27
Laboratory Materials and Techniques

1. A	2. B	3. D	4. C	5. B
6. B	7. D	8. B	9. B	10. A
11. D	12. A	13. B	14. C	15. B
16. B	17. B	18. A	19. C	20. C

CHAPTER 28
Advanced Chairside Functions

1. B	2. B	3. C	4. B	5. C
6. C	7. D	8. B	9. B	10. A
11. C	12. A	13. D	14. A	15. D
16. B	17. A	18. B	19. B	20. B
21. C	22. A	23. B	24. B	

CHAPTER 29
Dental Office Management

1. D	2. B	3. B	4. C	5. B
6. A	7. B	8. C	9. C	10. B
11. B	12. A	13. D	14. B	15. C
16. D	17. A			

CHAPTER 30
Employment Strategies

1. C	2. C	3. B	4. D	5. D
6. C	7. D	8. E	9. B	10. C
11. A	12. D	13. B	14. B	

CHAPTER 31
Ethics and Jurisprudence

1. C	2. D	3. B	4. B	5. A
6. C	7. D	8. A	9. B	10. A
11. D	12. C	13. B	14. D	15. C
16. D	17. C	18. C	19. C	20. A
21. C	22. C			